Osteoporosis

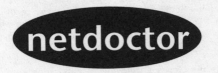

Series Editor
Dr Dan Rutherford
www.netdoctor.co.uk

Hodder & Stoughton
LONDON SYDNEY AUCKLAND

Copyright © 2004 by NetDoctor.co.uk
Illustrations copyright © 2004 by Amanda Williams

First published in Great Britain in 2004

The right of NetDoctor.co.uk to be identified as the Author of the Work has been asserted by them in accordance with the Copyright, Designs and Patents Act 1988.

10 9 8 7 6 5 4 3 2 1

British Library Cataloguing in Publication Data
A record for this book is available from the British Library

ISBN 0 340 86266 1

Typeset in Garamond by Avon DataSet Ltd,
Bidford-on-Avon, Warwickshire

Printed and bound in Great Britain by
Bookmarque Ltd, Croydon, Surrey

The paper and board used in this paperback are natural recyclable products made from wood grown in sustainable forests. The manufacturing processes conform to the environmental regulations of the country of origin.

Hodder & Stoughton
A Division of Hodder Headline Ltd
338 Euston Road
London NW1 3BH
www.madaboutbooks.com

Osteoporosis

Contents

Foreword

Osteoporosis, the brittle bone condition of adults, is a public health nightmare of global proportions. With increasing longevity this problem is likely to increase, including in developing countries such as in Asia and South America. In the UK it causes some 200,000 fractures every year, the cost of which to the NHS is approaching £2 billion per annum. Fortunately, recent years have seen rapid medical advances in diagnosis with newer imaging techniques and, more importantly, effective medications now available.

We can all also do a lot more to help ourselves, particularly from the point of view of prevention, as lifestyle factors are very important. Someone who has already had a fracture carries a much higher risk of a further fracture, but even so there is still scope to follow the right sort of advice and treatment to prevent further fractures. We have been promoting patient and public education and self-help training over the years in rheumatology but there is an even greater role for such 'expert patient' philosophy in managing osteoporosis.

This handbook for patients will provide all the necessary background and information about who is at risk, how to seek advice and help oneself, and what treatments are available. It will be equally valuable to nurses, trainee doctors and even general practitioners as it is presented in a succinct form.

The World Health Organisation has designated this decade as the decade for 'Bone and Joint Disorders'. With the new NHS Plan, a newer ethos and increasing public awareness, this is a very timely publication on a very important topic. It is my belief that every reader will find plenty of helpful information in this handbook on which he or she can take some action, rather than being a passive recipient of advice from health care professionals.

Dr Badal Pal MD, FRCP, D.Med Rhab
Consultant Rheumatologist and Honorary Lecturer
University of Manchester
South Manchester University Hospitals

Acknowledgements

I'm pleased to acknowledge the invaluable help of Dr Badal Pal, Consultant Rheumatologist from Withington Hospital in Manchester, who reviewed the contents of this book and made several helpful suffestions. Not for the first time has he pitched in with his time and enthusiasm despite a busy workload of his own.

Thanks are again gratefully extended to the team at Hodder & Stoughton who do all the behind-the-scenes work that ensures this book series continues to grow, Julie Hatherall, Judith Longman, Patrick Knowles and Amanda Williams in particular.

Sarah Mitchell, Research Physiotherapist at Glasgow Royal Infirmary, kindly provided details of the work she and her colleagues have done on physiotherapy guidelines in osteoporosis and I thank them too for allowing me to include their home exercise plan in the appendix.

Dr Douglas Smith, Consultant Radiologist in Fife, provided me with information on bone density scanning, for which I am very grateful.

Great care is taken to ensure that the information presented here is accurate and if any error still exists then the responsibility is mine. Please let me know if you spot any mistakes or have any suggestions for improving these books. I can be contacted at d.rutherford@netdoctor.co.uk

Dr Dan Rutherford
Medical Director
www.netdoctor.co.uk

Chapter 1

Osteoporosis – a Hidden Hazard

Despite its considerable importance osteoporosis, the 'weak bone' condition of adults, has only recently begun to attract the amount of attention it deserves from medical research and the health services. For a very long time we've been living with the consequences of osteoporosis, notably a steadily increasing number of middle-aged to older people with broken bones, and have not been doing an awful lot about it. There is still much that we do not understand about the condition, including the best ways to stop it happening in the first place, but much of what we do know is not yet widely enough publicised. Many thousands of people who could benefit from this information are currently not doing so. Just as bad is the excessive amount of confusing or unsound advice that exists around the subject. Our intention with this short book is to provide an easily readable but accurate summary of what happens to our bones as we get older, how to keep them as strong as possible and what needs to be done when they become weakened.

The impact of osteoporosis

It is self-evident that breaking (or *fracturing*) a bone causes a lot of pain and inconvenience to the individual concerned. Maybe too there is no such thing as a 'minor' fracture – a tiny crack in a finger bone may still be enough to hamper you considerably if you are a typist or a professional musician. However, the majority of bone fractures in young people are the result of fairly significant trauma and their powers of healing are rapid. In the older adults who get fractures due to osteoporosis many of the breaks occur with very minor trauma, such as a stumble or even a sneeze. Often there is no history of injury at all, as when a slowly developing forward stoop and loss of height due to osteoporosis of the spine occurs over several years.

Osteoporosis-related fractures are estimated to affect 30 per cent of women and 12 per cent of men at some time in their lives. One of the commonest such fractures is that of the hip – a serious injury with marked consequences not only for mobility but also for mortality. At any one time people with hip fractures occupy 20 per cent of all orthopaedic hospital beds in the UK. Six months after fracturing a hip only one third of people will be fully mobile and 10–20 per cent of people may die from the consequences of the fracture. The estimated annual cost of treating all fractures caused through osteoporosis is £1.6 billion in the UK alone. These sobering statistics surely underline the need for us to be looking at osteoporosis with as much concern as we already do with conditions like coronary artery disease and cancer.

Improving the care for osteoporosis

At present the majority of people who have osteoporosis are not known to have the condition prior to breaking a bone. Osteoporosis is an under-recognised condition, which is partly because in the UK we have not developed an organised approach to detecting it. As a result we do not yet consistently seek people at high risk of getting a fracture and offer them appropriate advice or treatment to reduce their risk. Even among the people who have had a fracture due to osteoporosis many do not receive follow-up treatment to help reduce their chance of getting another one.

There are very wide variations between the different regions of the UK in the quality and quantity of effort put in to detecting and treating osteoporosis and there are further divisions in the quality of care delivered to people from different social groups. For example, in a recent study carried out in Glasgow people from the most deprived areas were eight times less likely to be referred for the tests to detect osteoporosis than those from the most affluent areas.

There is, however, some good news too. The government has recognised the deficiencies that exist in osteoporosis management nationally and in 2002 accepted 'A Primary Care Strategy for Osteoporosis and Falls', published by the National Osteoporosis Society, which sets out the standards for osteoporosis care that ought to be achieved by Primary Care Organisations (see appendix A). As a result more funding is slowly coming through to expand the necessary services, such as bone scanning machines to diagnose osteoporosis, and the approach to the condition at GP and hospital level is becoming more co-ordinated.

Out of sight, out of mind

The main problem with osteoporosis is that it increases the risk of breaking a bone in a fall. Generally speaking, however, people with osteoporosis do not look any different from those with normal bone strength. Not everyone who breaks a bone in an apparently minor injury suffers from osteoporosis, even in the older age groups, nor does osteoporosis itself cause falls to occur. Someone who has quite marked osteoporosis but who never breaks a bone might remain completely unaware that they have the condition. This hidden nature of osteoporosis is of course one of the main reasons we have been neglecting it. Also, there has been too much readiness on the part of everyone to accept that when you get older you get frailer, are more prone to falls and that you break bones more easily. We've almost been agreeing that breaking a bone is a normal risk if you live long enough.

There is some truth in this, and one can't hold back the tide of time, but many older people have normal or above average bone strength whereas others the same age or younger may have osteoporosis. Osteoporosis is not inevitable with age and there is a great deal that the individual can do to reduce her or his chances of bone weakening.

Better awareness of osteoporosis among the general population and among health professionals will reduce the numbers of people getting osteoporosis and will improve our ability to pick up the condition at an earlier stage in those who do get it. There are now many treatments that can help bones to recover their strength but we need to target them better to the people who will benefit most from them. We'll be more specific later about who those people are.

Fragility, falls and fractures

Although most people with fractures recover well the outcome for others, as we've just seen, can be very serious indeed. Really there are three factors at play in deciding what happens to anyone with osteoporosis:

1 **Bone strength**, or fragility, is what we will be concentrating on in this book. The weaker someone's bones are then the greater is their risk of fracture when injured.

2 **The risk of falling**. A great many factors influence an individual's risk of falling, including their general medical condition and the hazards around them in the home and elsewhere. Tackling the many complex issues that are important in falls is already one of the major tasks of the health service and it will become increasingly important as the number of older people in the population increases.

3 **The type of injury**. Bones are good at resisting pressure applied along their length but are less able to resist force applied to the side. Whether a bone will break when it is struck therefore also depends on the angle at which the blow meets the bone. Chance can therefore play a big part in whether anyone, young or old, breaks a bone in a particular injury and not much can be done about luck. However, there are some ways and means of protecting against some injuries, such as hip fracture, should a fall occur, and we'll mention some.

Fragility, fall risk and the nature of the injury are like the three legs of a tripod. Take away any one leg and the tripod will fall. Reinforce all three legs and you will have a much-reduced chance of problems developing. Even if we had completely effective treatment that could make weak bones as strong as new, it would still be necessary to look at the causes of falls and at what can be done to minimise the impact of certain types of fall.

It makes all the difference to understanding osteoporosis and its treatment if one knows a bit about what makes bones 'tick', which is the subject of the next chapter.

Key Points

- Osteoporosis is an under-recognised condition and the majority of people with it are diagnosed only after they have suffered a bone fracture.
- Osteoporosis-related fractures are estimated to affect 30 per cent of women and 12 per cent of men at some time in their lives.
- The estimated annual cost of treating all fractures caused through osteoporosis is £1.6 billion in the UK alone.
- Osteoporosis is not inevitable with age and there is a great deal that the individual can do to reduce her or his chances of bone weakening.
- Bone fragility, fall risk and the nature of the injury are the factors that determine the outcome for someone with osteoporosis.

Chapter 2

The Private Life of Bones

We commonly think of bones as being dry and inert even in life. We don't generally credit them with being other than the internal scaffold that stops us collapsing in a heap. In fact, bone is highly active, living tissue constantly adapting to the stresses put upon it from body weight and the pull of muscles. Even as you read this book your bones will, ever so slightly, be changing to accommodate the mechanical stress put upon them.

Load-bearing exercise is one of the strongest stimuli that encourage bone to build up strength. The bones of a heavy manual labourer are stronger and thicker than those of a sedentary person of the same age, because they have adapted to be so. This is why exercise is one of the mainstays of the prevention and treatment of osteoporosis.

Hardly an everyday example, but nonetheless a dramatic one, is the rapid loss of bone observed in astronauts spending prolonged times in zero gravity. Within a few weeks they can lose massive amounts of their bone mass and strength unless regular load-bearing exercise is undertaken. A more common, terrestrial, example is the loss of strength of bone that can occur when a broken leg is encased in plaster for some time and the person has to bear weight only on the good leg. The plaster ensures that the ends of the break are kept in alignment during the healing process but the enforced inactivity in the broken leg can also cause a general loss of bone (and muscle) strength. This will normally recover quickly when the fracture is healed and normal activities are resumed. The phrase 'use it or lose it' applies very much to the bones.

If one takes a look at the detailed structure of bone one can see how it is that this constant re-modelling process occurs.

Bone structure

THE MAIN TYPES OF BONE

Taking a typical bone such as the femur (upper leg bone) and cutting it along its length shows a basic structure like that shown in figure 1. There is an outer shell of very hard bone (called 'cortical' bone) while in the middle space there is a honeycomb structure (called 'trabecular' or 'spongy' bone). Also, within the centre of the bone, is the bone marrow, a jelly-like substance that is the site of origin of the cells of the blood. The proportions of cortical and spongy bone vary in different parts of the skeleton depending on the loads that the particular area of bone has to cope with. Generally speaking cortical bone is the most abundant in the skeleton (about 80 per cent) and forms the dense outer shell of all bones. Cortical bone is very strong in resisting compression, which makes it suitable for carrying weight along its length; hence it forms the shafts of the long bones of the limbs. Because of its density cortical bone can withstand some bone loss, as in osteoporosis, without too much loss of strength.

Figure 1: Structure of femur

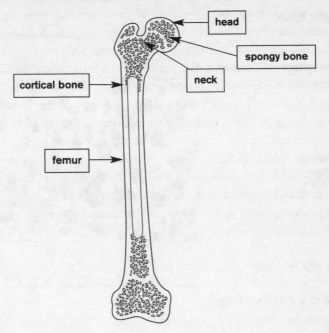

Trabecular or spongy bone is suited to forming complex shapes, thus for example it is predominant in the top part of the femur and within the ball of the hip joint. The honeycomb structure gives the maximum amount of strength for the least amount of weight but it is also more vulnerable to weakening in osteoporosis. Figure 2 shows the differences between normal and osteoporotic bone. In normal bone the lattice framework of central spongy bone is dense and strong and the outer cortical bone is thick. In osteoporotic bone the spongy bone becomes much finer and the cortical bone thins out. Spongy bone forms much of the type of bone found in the neck of the femur, at the wrist and within the vertebrae, which are also the most common sites of fracture in osteoporosis (figure 3).

Figure 2: Normal and osteoporotic bone structures

NORMAL BONE

bone surface →

internal meshwork of bone →

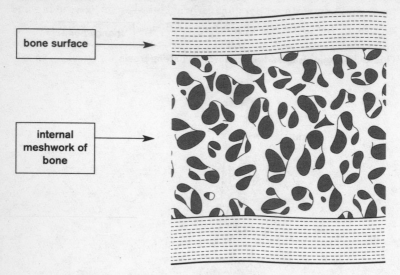

OSTEOPOROTIC BONE

thinner, weaker lattice of bone →

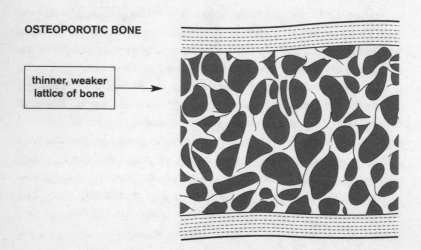

The main finding in osteoporosis is a drop in the amount of both types of bone at all sites throughout the skeleton. It is this loss of bone mass, and hence strength, particularly in critical areas like the hip and the spine, that gives rise to the increased likelihood of fractures.

Figure 3: Common sites for fractures in osteoporosis

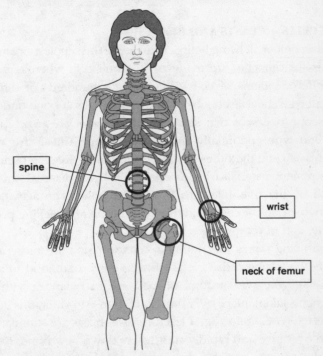

CHEMICAL MAKE-UP OF BONES

Bone is made up of fibres of a protein called collagen, on top of which are deposited several types of salts made from calcium and phosphate. By weight about 30 per cent of bone is collagen and 70 per cent salts. Individual fibres of collagen are extremely narrow but they exist in the millions, laid out a bit like the strands of a rope and aligned in the directions of the main forces acting on the bones. The salts exist in the form of minute crystals, locked on to the collagen fibres and bound to their neighbours. Collagen is a flexible protein, which is strong and resists stretching. The salt crystals bound to it and to each other resist compression and the combination gives bone its necessary physical properties.

BONE CELLS – 'CLASTS AND BLASTS'

The basic unit of all living beings is the cell. The simplest organisms, such as the amoeba, are made of just one cell, whereas human beings have billions of cells, divided into hundreds of different types all with specialised jobs to do. If one looks at bone under the microscope one sees that scattered throughout are two types of cell. One type continually makes new bone (these are called 'osteoblasts') and the other group continuously dissolve bone into its component materials (the 'osteoclasts'). These materials are then re-used by the osteoblasts to form new bone. The activities of these two groups of cell are at the heart of the remodelling process of bone, and of osteoporosis.

In growing bones the building cells ('blasts') are more active than the dissolving cells ('clasts') but in early adulthood to about middle age the two groups of cell are in balance, with fine adjustments taking place over time in response to variations in load such as exercise. Following a fracture osteoblasts are stimulated to go into overdrive and rapidly start to lay down new bone. Exactly what the triggers are that boost osteoblasts into such activity is not completely understood but physical stress at the fracture site is one of them. Orthopaedic surgeons, when repairing more complicated fractures in weight-bearing bones, regularly use this knowledge to speed up healing. By fixing the two sides of the break with splints that still allow a tiny amount of movement of the broken ends the rate of new bone formation is stimulated to increase. One also sees the remodelling process speeded up when a fracture of a load-bearing bone heals with the bone fragments slightly out of alignment. Not only is more bone deposited on the side of the break that has the most stress to carry but also over a longer period of time re-shaping of the break can occur. In young people without too much misalignment of the break to start with the eventual re-modelling may be nearly perfect – an invisible mend.

Bone is therefore far from static or inert – it is always on the go. It is estimated that about 10 per cent of an adult's bones are re-modelled every year – so in effect we get a new skeleton every 10 years! In older age the re-modelling process is much slower and the balance between the osteoblasts and osteoclasts changes slowly in favour of bone loss. We'll get to this in more detail shortly but first a few words are needed about calcium and vitamin D.

Calcium and vitamin D

CALCIUM

Calcium is an extremely important element used within a wide range of processes in the body. The contraction of muscles, conduction of impulses along the nerves, the normal process of blood clotting and many more actions are dependent on the body having ready access to calcium. The level of calcium within the blood and within the tissues is normally controlled very precisely by a complex process that, fortunately, it is not necessary to cover in great detail here! Suffice to say that it involves the control of how much calcium is absorbed by the digestive system from our food, how much we release via the kidneys into our urine and, particularly, the control of calcium in and out of bones. Almost 99 per cent of the total amount of calcium in our body is held within the skeleton. When the body requires more calcium it is drawn from the bone bank. In times of plenty the calcium is redeposited.

We get all of the calcium we need from our diet, but absorption of calcium from the digestive system is not very efficient. It is therefore important to maintain a good intake of calcium throughout life, and not just in our youth. When dietary intake is inadequate calcium is taken from the bones, weakening them. Some more information on dietary calcium intake is provided in chapter 6.

VITAMIN D

One of the main controlling influences on calcium in the body is vitamin D. Vitamin D increases the efficiency of the digestive system in absorbing calcium from the diet and it also stimulates calcium to go into the bones. A good intake of vitamin D is essential for bone health in everyone, and a lack of this vitamin can be a contributing factor in the development of osteoporosis. Elderly people, especially those who are sedentary or are in residential care, may have a low dietary intake of vitamin D and/or calcium and therefore may benefit from taking a supplement (chapter 8).

Strictly speaking vitamin D, in the form that is present in our diet, is not the active form of the vitamin used by the body. Instead vitamin D is converted into the active form by several complex chemical changes, first using the energy of sunlight on the skin, then by changes carried out by the liver and finally by reactions within the kidneys. It is not important to know the details, except to know that a straightforward lack of exposure to sunshine can be a cause of vitamin D deficiency.

Fortunately the active form of vitamin D is available as a medication or dietary supplement, so it is very easy to correct a deficiency. Later we'll be more specific about what constitutes the essentials of a diet for healthy bones.

These details are enough to understand the basics of how bone 'works' although there is a lot that has been left out from this description. There are other hormones with important effects on bones and calcium control, notably parathyroid hormone and calcitonin. Parathyroid hormone is produced by the 'parathyroid glands'. These are small pieces of tissue, just a few millimetres across, located behind the thyroid gland, which is situated in the front of the neck, below the 'Adam's apple'. Calcitonin is produced from cells within the thyroid gland. Abnormalities of production of these hormones do not cause osteoporosis although they can cause changes in the levels of calcium in the blood and some other bone conditions. Calcitonin can be used as a treatment for osteoporosis in some people (chapter 8).

Key Points

- Bone is highly active, living tissue constantly adapting to the stresses put upon it from body weight and the pull of the muscles.
- There are two main types of bone. Cortical bone is very dense and forms the outer shell of most bones. Trabecular, or spongy, bone forms the honeycomb structure within bone and is more prone to weakening in osteoporosis.
- Spongy bone forms much of the type of bone found in the neck of the femur, at the wrist and within the vertebrae, which are also the most common sites of fracture in osteoporosis.
- There are two types of cell active within bone. One type continually makes new bone (osteoblasts) and the other group continuously dissolves bone into its component materials for re-use (osteoclasts).
- The balance between the activity of the osteoblasts and osteoclasts is what makes it possible for bone to adapt to changes in load, such as body weight and muscle action, and is also at the heart of osteoporosis.

Chapter 3

Bone Mass

It should now be clear that there is a subtle, slowly acting process within bone that adapts it for the work it has to do. In the early years of life and up until we are between 20 and 30 years old the amount of bone within a healthy person's body steadily increases. Although we stop getting any taller in our late teens our bones go on getting thicker for several more years. Experts refer to the total amount of bone in the body as 'bone mass' and we therefore reach *peak bone mass* in our third decade, as illustrated in figure 4.

Figure 4 also shows that after remaining high for about 10 years it is normal for bone mass to fall. This happens to everyone, but not equally. Overall, the most important factor that influences the rate of fall of bone mass in later life is gender. The average older woman loses more bone mass than the average older man.

Figure 4: Peak bone mass with age (general)

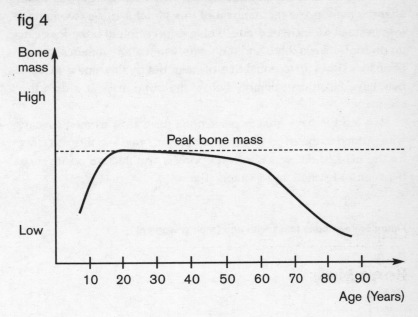

fig 4

Bones and oestrogen

Oestrogen is one of the two main 'female hormones', the other being progesterone. Produced by the ovaries the cyclical swings in production of these two hormones (also called the female sex hormones) are responsible for the changes of the menstrual cycle. At puberty the awakening of the ovaries and production of oestrogen and progesterone are what drives the development of the adult female body. At the other end of a woman's reproductive years the decline in output of female sex hormones is what causes the eventual cessation of periods – the menopause. The average age at which a woman goes through the menopause is 51 (with a normal range of about five years either side of this).

The relevance to bone strength is that oestrogen stimulates the bone-forming cells (osteoblasts), so when oestrogen levels drop after the menopause the removal of this stimulus causes women to lose bone at an increased rate. This period of rapid bone loss can go on for between three and ten years. Thereafter women's rate of bone loss slows up to equal that of men, but by this time a woman may have fallen considerably below the bone mass of a man the same age.

Men tend to have greater peak bone mass than women to start with. Added to the effect of postmenopausal bone loss this accounts for the marked difference in osteoporosis and fracture occurrence between older men and women (figure 5).

Figure 5: Peak bone mass with age (men v. women)

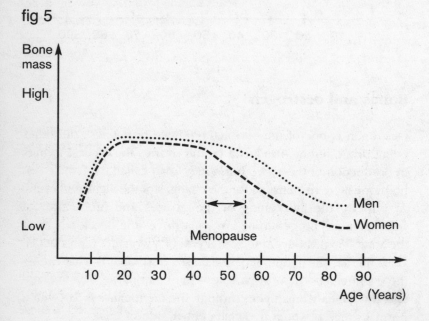

fig 5

Bone mass in men

Most discussions and explanations concerning osteoporosis focus on the impact of the condition in women. This is justifiable in terms of the numbers of people affected but it is wrong to think of osteoporosis as a strictly female condition. We've already seen that osteoporosis in general is under-recognised and inadequately treated but in men these problems are even worse than they are in women.

Men do develop osteoporosis and show an increased rate of osteoporotic hip fractures after the age of about 70, similar to the increase shown by women five to ten years younger. Men do not of course experience the recognisable hormone shift represented by the menopause in women, but they do experience a steady drop in output of testosterone (the 'male hormone') by the testes as they get older. Like oestrogen in women, testosterone has a protective effect on bone. More detail on the diagnosis and treatment of osteoporosis in men is given in chapter 9.

What is 'normal' bone mass?

We've seen that it is normal for bone mass to fluctuate throughout life and that there are differences in bone mass between men and women. Defining when bones are abnormally weak therefore has to take account of what is normal for the two sexes and the different age groups and so to some extent is a mathematical exercise. Modern bone scanning devices (about which there is more in chapter 5) can measure the density of bones and have allowed doctors to build up a range of readings across large numbers of people that set the range for 'normal' bone strength. Osteoporosis can therefore be said to be present if a person's bone density measurement is significantly low compared to these standards.

Range of normal

A tiny bit of mathematics will help to make sense of what a bone strength measurement actually means. Figure 6 shows the result you would get if you measured the height of a large number of people in a normal population and plotted them on a graph. A characteristic bell shape would result, showing that most people are at or about the middle of the height range and there are fewer people who are either very tall or very short. This sort of curve is typical when making many sorts of biological measurement. You would get a similar graph if, for example, you measured blood pressure, or weight. You also get this shape of curve if you measure bone mass from a large group of people the same sex and age.

Figure 6: Distribution of height in the population

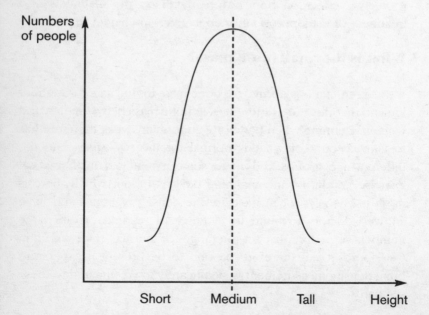

A mathematical calculation that we can thankfully skip over is then used to define a range either side of the middle that includes about 95 per cent of all people measured. This is illustrated in figure 7 as the shaded area. This is defined as the normal range for bone mass. In other words if your bone mass is anywhere within the shaded area, it is deemed to be within the normal range. Someone with a bone mass to the left of the lower range is below normal, and is said to have osteoporosis.

Figure 7: Definition of 'normal' bone mass

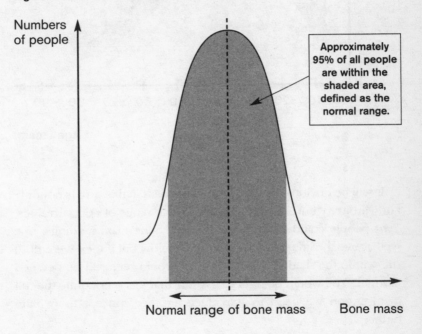

We can take this information and re-draw it to show a graph familiar from before. Figure 8 is the same as figure 4, indicating the general pattern of bone mass as it varies throughout life. This time, however, a shaded zone has been added which marks the range of normal either side of the middle.

Figure 8: Range of normal bone mass (or BMD – bone mineral density) with age

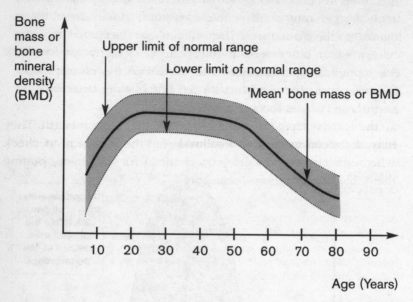

It will be obvious that defining bone mass in this way is not only fairly arbitrary but also that it gives a wide range of normal values. Two people could have quite different bone mass readings, one well above the line and the other well below but if they were both still within the shaded zone then they would both still be deemed 'normal'. You would be right to assume that this is not quite the full picture, and we need to introduce another concept to explain further.

Osteopenia

Osteopenia is this extra concept and it means 'slightly weak bones' (from the Greek words for bone – *osteon* and poverty – *penia*).

Osteopenia is again defined with the help of statistics, the details of which it is not necessary to know. In practical terms people with a bone mass in approximately the lower third of the normal range are said to have osteopenia. The significance of osteopenia is not entirely clear but is best thought of as a risk factor for the development of osteoporosis in the future. People with osteopenia will not necessarily need to take the sort of drug treatments for osteoporosis that we'll cover later but they do need to take seriously all the lifestyle changes that can improve their bone strength. They may also need more careful follow-up in the long term to check whether their bone strength has changed for the worse, putting them into the osteoporosis category.

Three positions are marked on figure 9 to illustrate these points. Each represents the bone mass of one of three women aged 60.

Figure 9: BMD readings on three 60-year-old individuals with normal BMD, osteopenia and osteoporosis

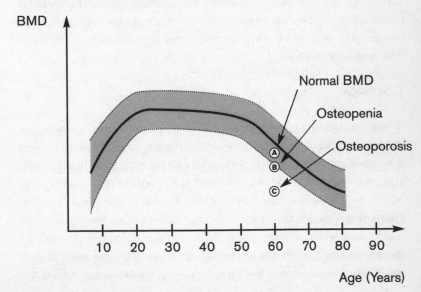

Point A is just below the mid-line but is well within the shaded area. This person's bone mass is therefore normal. Point B is someone with osteopenia, showing a bone density that is within the lower part of the normal range. Point C is the bone density of a woman with definite osteoporosis, with a reading below the lower range of normal.

Bone mass and bone density

Although osteoporosis is the condition in which the total mass of bone in the body is low we do not have practical ways of measuring total body bone mass. Instead we have machines (described in the next chapter) that measure the next best thing, which is bone density. Bone density, or bone mineral density (BMD) to give it its full title, is the amount of bone present within a given volume of space. In real life, therefore, bone mass is assessed by measuring BMD at specific sites, such as the wrist or spine, for which a large number of readings from the general population are already known. By comparing one with the other we get the picture of whether someone has normal, reduced or low bone strength.

T scores

If the preceding paragraphs have provided you with more information than you can presently digest, don't worry – most doctors don't need to carry around these facts in their head either! The main point of going over this area is to confirm that osteoporosis is not such a definite medical condition as it might initially seem. There is no black and white dividing line between strong, healthy bones and weak, fragile ones. Bone strength is more a series of shades of grey, with osteoporosis representing one end of that spectrum. (We have not touched at all on conditions in which the bones become very dense. These do exist but they are rare and are outside the scope of this book.)

A useful shorthand way of expressing the results of a bone density measurement is a figure known as the T score. The T score is based on exactly the same principles as we've already covered earlier in this chapter and represents how far below the average a person's bone mineral density (BMD) reading is. The T score is a number above (+) or below (−) zero. Numbers below zero indicate lower than average bone density, thus:

- T score 0 to −1 = normal range
- T score −1 to −2.5 = osteopenia
- T score less than −2.5 = osteoporosis

The T score is often the result that will be the one most looked for by the doctor when he or she receives the result of a bone density test on a patient. Now you too know what it means! Definitions of osteoporosis based on the T score have arisen from research carried out on female populations rather than male. Experts, however, apply the same T score criteria to men as for women.

Low impact fractures

A person can also be deemed to have osteoporosis if they have suffered a fracture too easily, i.e. a 'low impact' or 'low trauma' or 'osteoporotic' fracture. This is something of a circular definition but nonetheless identifying people who have osteoporosis after they have suffered the consequences and concentrating upon them efforts at prevention does reduce the chance of their suffering another fracture later.

A low trauma fracture is one that occurs from a fall from standing height or less and fractures of the hip, wrist or forearm can be categorised in this way fairly easily. It is more difficult to do so for the spine as many spinal fractures occur out of the blue and are not related to falls – often they are not even accompanied by much pain.

The occurrence of a low impact fracture should trigger alarm bells that the person has established osteoporosis. Often that will best be confirmed by then checking with a bone density test. Sometimes the evidence that a person has osteoporosis is so clear that a BMD test is unnecessary and treatment for osteoporosis can be started right away.

Other factors affecting bone mass

Understanding what affects bone mass underpins much of what we know about osteoporosis, but that is not to say we entirely understand the process. However, if one takes large numbers of people and looks at what is common to those who develop osteoporosis versus those who do not, several patterns, or 'risk factors', emerge.

Generally speaking, people with osteoporosis:

- are women;
- are elderly;
- have a history of a previous fracture;
- have a family history of osteoporosis;
- are of low body weight;
- are physically inactive (see below);
- have a reduced intake of calcium in the diet;
- who are women, were late to start having periods and/or they reached the menopause at a young age (under 45 years old);
- smoke;
- have a raised alcohol intake.

Although people with many risk factors are more likely to get osteoporosis than those with few or none it is not possible to predict osteoporosis with any certainty in an individual from these factors alone. As we've just pointed out, men also get osteoporosis, not just women. So too do people who are not yet elderly. Having a history of previous fracture occurring after relatively minor injury (a 'low trauma' fracture) is strongly associated with osteoporosis, but the condition was present when the person had their first fall and fracture too, at which time they had no prior history. So the value of risk factors is largely to show the overall picture and to illustrate some of the things we can do to prevent osteoporosis. Of course not all are modifiable – we can't stop ourselves aging or change our gender or family history.

EXTREME EXERCISE
The effect of regular load-bearing exercise is to increase bone strength but there is an exception in the case of the small percentage of women who are elite athletes. Some such women who train to very high levels of fitness are underweight and they achieve a low peak bone mass in young adulthood. Over-training also tends to stop their periods occurring, so they have less oestrogen stimulation of their bones. These problems are, however, experienced only by a very small minority of women. The vast majority of women who exercise to keep fit, including those who do so to quite a high level, do not need to be concerned that they are storing up trouble for their bones later in life – quite the reverse.

Steroids and osteoporosis

A small number of prescription medicines are known to accelerate the rate of bone loss. By far the commonest of these are the drugs known as 'steroids'. Steroids are widely used in the medical treatment of many conditions such as some types of arthritis and the 'connective tissue diseases' (e.g. rheumatoid arthritis and systemic lupus erythematosus, or SLE). Asthma sufferers often require steroid inhalers for treatment but the dose of steroid taken into the body from inhalers is not sufficient to cause bone weakening. However, many people with more severe asthma need to take steroid tablets or injections, in which case the dose is much higher. Although asthma is a common example there are several other medical conditions in which long-term use of oral steroids is necessary.

Short courses of steroids, up to a few weeks, do not have any significant impact on bone strength but when they need to be taken for longer periods of time then they can cause bone weakening, because steroids stimulate the bone-dissolving cells (osteoclasts) to become more active. Patients taking long-term steroids therefore need to be advised on also taking treatment to protect against bone loss (chapter 10).

Other 'secondary' causes of osteoporosis

'Secondary' osteoporosis means osteoporosis caused by some other illness or factor. Steroid drug therapy is the commonest cause of secondary osteoporosis. There are rare medical conditions in which the body's natural production of steroids is markedly increased and these can cause osteoporosis too. Osteoporosis is sometimes seen in people with alcoholism, partly because of the fact that their diet is often poor but also because a high alcohol intake appears to weaken the bones directly. Osteoporosis is also sometimes seen in association with diabetes and in people with an over-active thyroid gland.

A few drugs other than steroids can cause osteoporosis. Heparin is a 'blood thinning' medicine (anticoagulant) usually used in short courses such as after major operations, to reduce the likelihood of blood clots occurring. Such short-term use has no effect on bone strength. Rarely heparin is used for months at a time, for example in pregnancy when the mother has a high risk of developing clots due to the presence of other medical conditions. Osteoporosis has been observed following the use of heparin over many months.

Key Points

- Bone mass is the total amount of bone in the body.
- Peak bone mass is reached between the ages of 20 and 30 and thereafter begins to decline in all healthy people.
- Men tend to achieve a higher peak bone mass than women.
- Women have an increased rate of bone loss for between three and ten years following the menopause.
- Normal bone mass is defined by calculations based on large numbers of readings from the average population.
- Bone mineral density (BMD) is the amount of bone present within a given volume of space.
- The T score is a shorthand way of expressing bone mineral density. A T score less than −2.5 is the generally accepted level for diagnosing osteoporosis.
- A number of risk factors are associated with the development of osteoporosis. Generally speaking, people with the most risk factors are at the highest risk.

Chapter 4

Testing and Screening for Osteoporosis

Given that osteoporosis is such a big problem but that it is largely undetected it would seem to make a lot of sense that we should be trying to find people who have the condition, and offer them treatment. Similarly people who have osteopenia, if they knew about it soon enough, could make an informed choice to try hard to reverse the trend. The fact that we do not have an organised screening service for osteoporosis in the UK reflects many issues, and although a lack of funding is one of them it is by no means the only one. No other country in the world, including those that spend more on healthcare than the UK, has such a screening service either. Often we blame the under-funding of the NHS for all its deficiencies but even if we spent millions on putting bone scanners all over the country and could afford to offer such tests to virtually everyone in middle age or older we would still not have solved all the problems associated with osteoporosis screening.

The problems with osteoporosis screening

Screening for osteoporosis would be worthwhile if we knew that by doing so we could reduce the burden of illness to individuals and the costs to the health service of osteoporotic fractures. For that to be the case we would need to have effective treatment for osteoporosis that could be taken by the majority of people and which would halt the progress of the condition. As we'll see in the following chapters we do have treatment that fulfils some of these requirements, some in the form of lifestyle changes and others in the form of drugs. However, to be effective the treatments, whatever they may be, need to be kept going for a very long time. People most at risk of falls and fractures are over 80 years old. Screening for osteoporosis in people aged 50 or 60 therefore raises the problem of how long do you keep up with the treatment – 30 years? We do not yet have long-term experience of the more recent types of osteoporosis drug treatments to know if they are safe to take for such periods of time. Certainly many people already find that they have side effects that make them hard to take even for relatively short periods.

Furthermore, one of the most effective treatments for osteoporosis, hormone replacement therapy, is very much under the spotlight these days and few if any people will be well advised or willing to take HRT for several decades. Yet we know that as soon as HRT is stopped the bone protection it confers falls away.

Issues such as this are at the heart of present debates concerning osteoporosis screening. Because they raise difficult questions does not of course mean that we should throw up our hands and give up on the idea. Osteoporosis is a condition that undoubtedly requires action if we are to curtail the rise in people affected by it. Screening for it is not a straightforward issue and detecting low bone mass in people who are not yet elderly can give rise to some difficult choices.

The problems with bone density tests

When bone density tests give a very low result, indicating definite osteoporosis in need of treatment, then there is no doubting their usefulness. If bone density tests are done in an elderly population of people then quite a few people with osteoporosis will be detected as a result. The best use of screening would, however, be to detect these people 10 to 20 years earlier, when action to treat osteoporosis would have had considerably more impact. In the case of women this would be around the time of their menopause, and this is also the group within the population who are the most likely to be seeking advice on their osteoporosis risk from their doctor.

Bone density testing at the time of the menopause would, however, detect far fewer women with definite osteoporosis, simply because it is less common in younger women. Moreover, the level of bone density of an individual woman at the time of her menopause is actually a poor predictor of her eventual risk of suffering a bone fracture. One can see the dilemma. We have a condition that we know we need to do better at detecting, but the tools we have to detect it early are presently too crude and the available drug treatments have not been tested for extended periods of time.

The question is not so much how we screen for osteoporosis, as whether any form of screening is any use at all. This is a very big issue that is currently the subject of much research, and we are not going to be able to answer it completely here. What is perhaps the most important point to make clear is that this is an area where we do not yet have the required answers. It certainly will not transform the landscape of bone health if we rush into doing bone density tests on all and sundry without considering what we will do with the results. Random or indiscriminate use of bone density screening will pick up some of those people who have osteoporosis but it will miss most of them and will waste a lot of manpower and money in the process. Clearly we need to target our efforts more effectively, so that those at the highest risk get the earliest attention.

Risk scoring

It would be a great help if there were something like a reliable screening questionnaire that individuals could complete and which gave a score indicating that person's likelihood of developing osteoporosis. People with a high score could then go on to have further tests. Although several such 'risk score' tools have been tried out none has proved good enough for general use. Either they point out too many people needing more tests, which is not much help if the system is already struggling to cope with demand, or they provide false reassurance that someone's bone strength is probably fine, when in fact it is not. Some of these tools manage to have both faults at the same time!

So, who needs a bone scan?

The following categories of people need to consider themselves at the highest risk of having or developing osteoporosis, and until better screening procedures come along these are the people who ought to be going along to their doctor, if they have not already done so, to talk about osteoporosis testing:

1. PREVIOUS HISTORY OF FRACTURE

A previous history of fracture, especially if it is or could have been a low trauma fracture, is one of the most important pointers to the presence of osteoporosis. Too many people who suffer a low trauma fracture are still not being properly considered as potentially having osteoporosis and so are not receiving ideal care. This situation is beginning to change now for the better but there are still many gaps in the system. Certainly many people who sustained such fractures more than a few years ago will probably be still going around with their osteoporosis unnoticed. So a personal history of fracture, even if it is not recent, should be acted upon.

2. LOSS OF HEIGHT OR DEVELOPING A STOOP

Osteoporosis of the spine can cause a loss of height, which is considered significant if it is over 5cm compared with your young adult height. Alternatively, or additionally, a forward stoop of the spine may develop. Both of these are suggestive features of osteoporosis and merit further assessment by your doctor.

3. PEOPLE OVER 60

Osteoporosis is commoner in older people, and estimates in female populations show that within the age range 60–69 around 24 per cent of women have osteoporosis. This is certainly higher than the numbers of people in this age range who have been diagnosed with the condition. Age groups older than this of course have a higher likelihood of being osteoporotic. Younger age groups still contain people with osteoporosis but in much fewer numbers, and one has to make a judgement of the age band where a general policy of osteoporosis screening would be sufficiently worthwhile for large numbers of people to take part in it.

To undertake the routine screening (by bone density scans) of all individuals over the age of 60 would clearly be a massive exercise that is simply not feasible within our present resources, but this is not the best reason for discarding the idea. The National Osteoporosis Foundation in the USA recommended in 1998 that bone mineral density measurements should be done in all women aged over 65. At some point we in the UK will need to tackle the numbers problem too.

4. WOMEN WHO HAVE HAD AN EARLY MENOPAUSE

The average age of women at the menopause is 51 and those who go through the 'change of life' below the age of 45 are considered to have done so early. The drop in bone strength that accompanies the fall in oestrogen levels of the menopause has already been discussed. The earlier the menopause is experienced the sooner this fall in bone strength will start, unless the woman is given oestrogen-containing hormone replacement therapy (chapter 7). Hormone replacement therapy (HRT) of this type provides the same level of bone protection as the natural function of the ovaries but only so long as it is taken. As soon as it is stopped then bone strength starts to fall in postmenopausal women. As is also covered in chapter 7, HRT has become a controversial subject in the past year or two and many women who were taking it have stopped doing so. This may have some influence on the numbers of women developing osteoporosis in the years to come.

5. FAMILY HISTORY OF OSTEOPOROSIS

Population surveys of people who have a family history of osteoporosis show that they are likely to have lower than average bone density readings themselves. Such a family history might be quite difficult to establish bearing in mind that osteoporosis is often missed, but suggestive features would be a family member who had a low trauma fracture after the age of 50, or who developed the forward stoop of the 'dowager's hump' mentioned earlier. Some will of course have had a formal diagnosis based on bone density testing. The family history should be taken from as many near relatives as possible, and not just from the parents. It is important to include men as well as women in the history taking, as they are equally important.

Other factors

Several other factors can raise an individual's risk:

1. ETHNIC ORIGIN
White women have 2.5 times the risk of developing osteoporosis compared with women of Afro-Caribbean origin. (Asian women, particularly Muslims, living in the UK are at greater than average risk of being seriously deficient in vitamin D, which increases their risk of developing a different bone condition called osteomalacia.)

2. SMOKING
Bone density in men and women who smoke is less than in non-smokers and female smokers are at greater risk of hip fracture than non-smokers.

3. INADEQUATE EXERCISE
A sedentary lifestyle, including a history of such in adolescence, is associated with lower bone density in adulthood. Current exercise is associated with increased bone density. The fact that being inactive in one's youth can lead to long-term reduction in bone strength is one other important reason why we need to encourage

young people to take regular physical exercise. The good news for those who are now past the flush of youth, however, is that getting active helps not only your bones but every other important health-related issue as well.

4. LOW BODY WEIGHT

People who are unusually thin are more likely to develop osteoporosis, and the way to define 'thin-ness' is to measure the body mass index (BMI). The BMI is a simple mathematical formula that relates a person's weight to their height and therefore can be applied to any person, whether tall or short, and to both sexes.

To calculate a BMI, take the person's weight (in kilograms) and divide it by the square of their height (in metres). For example, an 80kg person of height 1.7 metres will have a BMI of $80/(1.7 \times 1.7) = 27.7 \text{kg/m}^2$. Someone who is 1.5 metres tall and weighs 47kg would have a BMI of $47/(1.5 \times 1.5) = 20.9 \text{ kg/m}^2$.

The ranges of BMI are:

- Normal   = 20–24.9
- Overweight   = 25–30
- Obese   = Over 30

People with a BMI of 21 or less have a higher rate of bone loss than those who are heavier, and obese people have lower rates of bone loss than those who are ideal weight. It is not known if a thin person who deliberately puts on a lot of weight will reduce their subsequent fracture risk. Obesity of course carries with it many other health hazards, so the message is clearly that keeping within the range of normal weight is good for your bones as well as your general health.

5. HIGH ALCOHOL CONSUMPTION

Historically the recommended maximum consumption of alcohol per week was 21 units for women and 28 units for men. High levels of alcohol intake (over 50 units per week in men, or 35 units in women) are definitely associated with osteoporosis, as well as all the other serious health risks that accompany alcoholism. It is possible that lower levels of alcohol consumption than this could still damage bone as well as be associated with other health problems such as raised blood pressure or diabetes. Many experts therefore now recommend lower safe limits of alcohol consumption of 21 units weekly for men and 14 units weekly for women.

A unit of alcohol is:

- 250ml (½ pint) of ordinary strength beer / lager
- 1 glass (125ml / 4 fl oz) of wine
- 1 pub measure of sherry / vermouth (1.5 fl oz)
- 1 pub measure of spirits (1.5 fl oz)

Action on risk factors

The above factors are the main ones associated with the development of osteoporosis. Secondary reasons, such as steroid therapy, are also important to include in this list. In the absence of a reliable 'risk-scoring' system it is not possible to put a value on these items, tot up the points and come up with a magic number that says you do or do not have osteoporosis. The best one can say is that the more of these items that apply to you, the greater is the threat of osteoporosis to you personally.

If many of these risk factors do apply to you then it does not automatically mean that your next move should be an anxious appointment at the doctor and insistence on seeing a bone expert. For many people the correct response will be to look at their present lifestyle and decide what moves they can make towards improving their bone strength.

The best person to initially advise you about the relevance of this information to yourself is your GP. If necessary he or she can either refer you to an osteoporosis exert for their opinion, or in many regions the GP can refer you directly for tests such as bone density scanning. Protocols to guide the correct use of tests such as bone density scanning are now commonplace across the UK and although they may vary a bit in the exact details the basic principles are the same. Usually these referral guidelines cover a selection of the main risk factors and omit those that are harder to quantify, such as the degree of exercise someone takes.

For example, a typical referral guideline could look like the following; the presence of one factor justifying the GP requesting a bone density scan:

- A woman over 50 who has had a low trauma fracture.
- Anyone taking oral steroid (prednisolone 5mg daily or greater for three or more months).
- A woman under 45 who has had an early menopause or removal of the ovaries.
- A woman who is around the menopause who also has any two of the following risk factors:
  - ☐ Smokes
  - ☐ Has a body mass index less than 21
  - ☐ Has a history in her mother of a hip fracture below 80 years of age
  - ☐ Drinks more than 35 units of alcohol weekly.
- A man with a high alcohol consumption of over 50 units of alcohol weekly.

Despite their limitations, bone mineral density measurements are the mainstay of osteoporosis diagnosis. The next chapter considers the practicalities of this test in more detail.

Key Points

- Although osteoporosis is under-diagnosed, population screening for it would not be straightforward, even if adequate funding were available.
- The people most likely to benefit from bone density screening are listed in this chapter.
- There are slight differences in local health trust policies across the UK that guide the referral of patients for bone density screening. These need to be discussed with your GP.

Chapter 5

Bone Density Testing

Diagnosing osteoporosis

X-RAYS

When an ordinary X-ray is taken and developed the film is a mixture of dark areas, where the X-rays have exposed the film, and light areas where the X-rays have been less able to get through. Dense tissues such as bone are harder for X-rays to penetrate, so they show up white on a dark background. Bones that are osteoporotic are easier for X-rays to pass through, so they can appear to be less white than normal bones. However, ordinary X-rays are not reliable as a means of diagnosing osteoporosis, for various technical reasons. The same fainter appearance of the bones can occur if the exposure of the film is too high. Conversely if the film is underexposed then the bones will look denser than they should. In any case as much as 30 per cent of bone mass needs to be lost before it shows up on ordinary X-rays, which is far too much. Modern digital X-ray machines no longer use film but instead use detectors that are sensitive to X-rays. Images obtained this way can be enhanced in different ways, which makes it easier to see fine details but even harder to suspect the presence of osteoporosis.

X-rays can, however, still be of some use. If an X-ray of the spine of an older person shows several areas of bone collapse within the vertebrae then, in the absence of a history of injury, the likely cause of such findings would be osteoporosis of the spine. Further tests can then be done to confirm this.

ULTRASOUND

High frequency sound waves have found many uses in medical investigation. The vast majority of women who have given birth within the past few decades will be familiar with the ultrasound scans that show the baby in the womb. Ultrasound scanners are a safe, painless and quick way of looking at structures within the body and can also be used to detect bone density. Essentially pulses of sound are sent through a bone such as the heel bone, which is easily accessible, and the speed of the sound waves through the heel indicates the density of the bones. The beauty of ultrasound is that it is very quick and cheap to do. The instruments are relatively inexpensive and are portable, so this method has understandably become quite popular; it is also used by private clinics offering osteoporosis screening. The main difficulty with ultrasound is that the results are highly dependent on the particular type of machine and the techniques used. It is not yet clear whether ultrasound is sufficiently reliable and accurate to use as a main tool for the diagnosis and monitoring of osteoporosis but there is much current research on it. One study in general practice that used heel ultrasound in addition to 'risk scoring' improved the ability to detect women who were shown to have osteoporosis by subsequent DXA scan (see below), and this is probably the best way in which to use ultrasound testing at the present time.

DXA SCANNING

Currently the gold standard for measuring bone density is the 'dual-energy X-ray absorpiometry' test, or 'DXA' scan for short. As the name implies, a DXA scan uses X-rays to determine the density of bone, but in a different way from X-ray photography. DXA scanning machines are expensive and need to be sited in one place but they give accurate and reproducible results. The amount of X-rays used in carrying out a DXA scan is extremely small and poses no hazard to health. The procedure is very simple, takes under 20 minutes and involves lying on your back on the couch that is part of the machine while the bone density reading is taken.

To increase the accuracy of the DXA scan at least two measurements are made at different sites of the body. Typically a measurement will be made of the spine and a hip. The results are printed as a graph showing the patient's bone density within the expected range for their age, much like figure 10. The machine also calculates the patient's T score.

The DXA test gives a 'stand-alone' result, i.e. the result is sufficient on its own to make the diagnosis of osteoporosis. This is in contrast to the ultrasound test, the result of which needs to be interpreted in the light of other risk factors and is not on its own good enough to diagnose osteoporosis.

Other tests

Other types of machine exist that are capable of measuring bone density but these are either not in common use or are still at the research stage.

Figure 10: DXA scanning and an example result

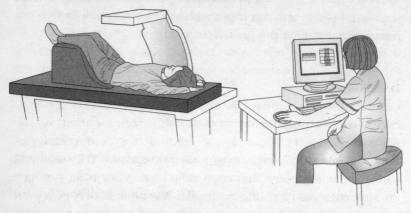

Example of a lumbar spine DXA report

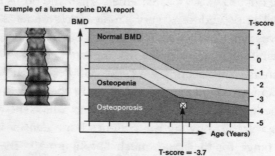

T-score = -3.7

Example of a hip DXA report

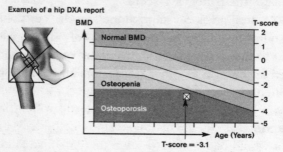

T-score = -3.1

Mrs Jane Smith
Age: 66
Height: 150cm
Weight: 49kg
Average T-score: -3.4
Diagnosis: osteoporosis

A completely different approach is to test the blood and urine for the presence of chemicals produced as a result of bone loss. Again these techniques are still largely in development. It is possible that a combination of new or emerging technologies will replace the DXA scan in due course but for the meantime this is the test we need to rely on.

Should bone scans be repeated?

A single bone scan is only a snapshot, giving a reading at one point in an individual's life. Bearing in mind the slow pace at which bone strength usually changes, a BMD reading will be valid for some time thereafter, but no one is exactly sure for how long. One of the other big questions in osteoporosis is therefore whether re-testing is necessary, and if so how often?

From the patient's point of view, given that DXA scanning is harmless, a repeat scan every so often for someone deemed at high risk of getting osteoporosis would provide reassurance that their bone strength is not ebbing away despite their best efforts to prevent it doing so. For those people taking treatment for osteoporosis repeated tests would show whether they were actually doing themselves any good by taking the tablets. It is probably true that if we had plenty of bone scanners then there would be less argument about repeat scanning. As we still haven't done a first scan on a large section of the population there is an understandable reluctance for anyone to recommend repeat scanning unless the result will have a direct bearing on treatment. An example might be a person with low BMD but who was still within the normal range (i.e. who has osteopenia). Repeat testing perhaps one to two years later would be justified to see if the BMD had fallen further, to a level at which osteoporosis drug treatment was necessary. Each person has to be judged on his or her own merits, so only a generalisation can be put here. The summary position about repeat scanning is therefore that it is not recommended except in special circumstances, such as when the result would directly influence the subsequent choice of treatment.

Key Points

- Bone density scanners are the only fully reliable technical means of diagnosing osteoporosis at the present time.
- There are several types of bone density scanning devices, but the most widely used is the dual-energy X-ray absorpiometry (DXA) scan.
- DXA scanning uses very low doses of X-ray radiation and is safe.
- Osteoporosis cannot be diagnosed by ordinary X-ray investigations.
- Ultrasound is already capable of suggesting osteoporosis and will probably become increasingly useful as it is technically improved, but currently should not be relied on as the sole test for osteoporosis.

Chapter 6

Prevention and Treatment of Osteoporosis: (a) Lifestyle and Self-help Measures

Exercise

Technology, in the form of motorised transport, has removed the need for us to expend much energy getting from A to B. We no longer have to forage for food – a glide along the aisles of the local supermarket is the closest we come to that activity now. Television and computer games allow us to occupy our minds without engaging our bodies. All of these activities run counter to the way we are designed to work in a biological sense and have been in the habit of living for thousands of years. The evidence supporting the health benefits of exercise is not in dispute. Exercise certainly protects against osteoporosis and reduces the risk of falls in older people but it also gives major reductions in coronary heart disease, blood pressure and cholesterol levels, lowers the occurrence of obesity, diabetes, cancer of the colon and breast and increases psychological well-being. Of all the stress-busting treatments that we undoubtedly need in this day and age, nothing is as effective or as good for you as a long walk.

Walking is in many ways the ideal form of exercise. It can be undertaken by most people and started at a modest level appropriate for someone who's been out of the exercise habit for a long time. It doesn't need expensive equipment and can be as social or as private as you want it to be. Brisk walking is good aerobic exercise that doesn't jar the joints too much and injuries when walking are rare. Cycling is also suitable for a wide range of people and can often be incorporated easily into daily living. Its benefits are amazing. Cycling for 25 miles per week was associated with a 50 per cent reduction in risk of dying from all causes over a 10-year follow-up period in one study.

The sorts of exercise that benefit people with osteoporosis are of two types:

1 Strength training – in which muscles are worked against a load. This needs to be targeted to specific muscle groups, such as, for example, those that move the hip joint.
2 Low impact weight bearing activity. Low impact weight bearing is defined as always having one foot on the floor. (High impact weight bearing has both feet off the floor, such as jumping, and is not suitable for people with established osteoporosis.)

Although some general principles of exercise can be set out it is preferable for anyone with osteoporosis or osteopenia to seek the advice of a physiotherapist before starting on an exercise programme. Physiotherapists are always keen to see people looking for such advice, as all too often they have to help people after fractures and would rather be helping to prevent them occurring. A referral from your GP is usually required for you to access the local physiotherapy service.

Guidelines of the Chartered Society of Physiotherapy

The professional guidelines produced by the Chartered Society of Physiotherapy for the management of osteoporosis (1999, appendix A) set out recommendations for the three groups of people who are likely to seek exercise advice in respect of their bone health:

1 Those with normal bone mass or osteopenia who wish to reduce their risk of getting osteoporosis later in life
2 Those with osteoporosis diagnosed on clinical grounds or on bone density testing but who have no history of fracture
3 Those with more severe osteoporosis, who usually have also sustained one or more fractures.

A) NORMAL OR LOW BONE MASS (OSTEOPENIC) GROUP
High impact exercise, such as skipping and jogging, is suitable for this group, at least for those who are used to exercising. Those not used to exercise or over 50 years old can work up from a low impact starting point such as step aerobics or intermittent jogging. The exercise programme needs to be built up steadily as strength and fitness improve.

B) OSTEOPOROTIC BUT NO FRACTURE
Maximum benefit appears to be gained from strength work that uses a high load but low number of repetitions, i.e. it is the

maximum load on the muscle that matters more than its endurance. This is combined with aerobic, low impact exercise.

C) SEVERE OSTEOPOROSIS OR A HISTORY OF FRACTURES

The main aim of exercise in this group of people is to minimise their risk of falling. Exercise will usually need to start from a low level but even seated exercise is helpful. Strength training can be done using body resistance to start with. Exercise in water (hydrotherapy), when available, is particularly suitable for people who have pain from a recent fracture, or who are frail or lack confidence in their mobility. Activities such as Tai Chi are good for improving balance.

A simple general home exercise plan is detailed in appendix C.

Modifiable risk factors

SMOKING

Stopping smoking benefits bone health, and just about every other aspect of health too. The raised risk of osteoporosis fades with time although it can be up to 10 years before it is the same as for a non-smoker. The reduction in risk of lung cancer takes the same or longer to occur in ex-smokers and never quite drops to equal a non-smoker's risk. The message is that it is never too late, or too soon, to stop smoking.

ALCOHOL

The health risks of alcohol excess extend well beyond the bones, but as alcohol is directly toxic to bone cells stopping drinking allows them to start the process of recovery.

WEIGHT

Underweight people have low bone mass. It is likely (although not proven) that someone who is underweight who corrects this towards normal will reduce his or her subsequent risk of developing osteoporosis.

Calcium intake

A good calcium intake is essential throughout life for healthy bones and there is good evidence that the adequacy of a child's diet at least partially determines their osteoporosis risk in adulthood. Although dairy products are high in calcium they are not the only source. Non-dairy food sources include:

- nuts and pulses (almonds, Brazil nuts, hazelnuts, sesame seeds);
- green leafy vegetables (broccoli, spinach, watercress, curly kale);
- dried fruits (apricots, dates, figs);
- fish (mackerel, pilchards, salmon, sardines);
- tofu and various calcium-fortified foods.

The usual recommended daily intake of calcium for adults over 50 is 700 milligrams but a combined analysis of medical research studies concluded that postmenopausal women should aim for a dietary intake of 1,000 milligrams daily. (This level of intake was associated with a 24 per cent reduction in the occurrence of hip fractures.) On average 250ml or half a pint of cow's milk contains 360 milligrams of calcium. Low-fat dairy products contain the same amount of calcium as higher fat varieties. A more detailed list of foods and their calcium content is in appendix D.

Calcium supplements can be bought and there are several types available on prescription if someone's dietary intake is low or marginal. Taking a supplement of calcium along with vitamin D may help frail elderly people. This type of supplement is safe but is best discussed with a doctor first (chapter 8).

Key Points

- Lifestyle-based actions are appropriate for everyone, both to prevent osteoporosis and to treat it.
- Regular exercise is essential and has a number of other health benefits. Advice can be obtained from a physiotherapist concerning the appropriate type and amount of exercise for an individual, and is advisable for those who already have osteoporosis.
- An adequate dietary intake of calcium and vitamin D is essential for bone health.
- Avoidable risk factors for osteoporosis include smoking and excess alcohol consumption.

Chapter 7

Prevention and Treatment of Osteoporosis: (b) Hormone Replacement Therapy (HRT)

HRT slows the rate at which bone is lost in women following the menopause and may even reverse the process of osteoporosis, at least temporarily. HRT is not the only drug treatment used in osteoporosis (the others are covered in the next chapter) but it is the longest established. HRT is also the subject of much controversy and debate at the present time, which is why it deserves a chapter on its own. (A fuller description of HRT and its roles are contained in the companion volume in this series, on the menopause.)

Strictly speaking HRT is licensed only to protect against the development of osteoporosis rather than as a treatment for established osteoporosis. In practical terms doctors prescribe it for both reasons.

What is hormone replacement therapy?

The use of hormones (oestrogen and progesterone-like medicines) to boost the fall in output of the menopausal ovaries is a treatment that has been around now for over 60 years. Early HRT experience with oestrogen replacement had the desired effect of relieving menopausal symptoms such as hot flushes, but it was discovered in the 1970s that women using it who still had their womb (i.e. they had not had it removed for some reason such as heavy bleeding) had an increased risk of developing cancer of the lining of the womb after some years of oestrogen use. The medical name for the lining of the womb is the endometrium; hence this type of cancer is called endometrial cancer. The reason was traced to the continuous stimulating effect of oestrogen upon the cells of the endometrium.

During the normal menstrual cycle oestrogen waxes and wanes and so too does progesterone. Oestrogen predominates in the first half of the cycle and progesterone in the second. In general terms cancer occurs when a cell runs out of control, duplicating repeatedly without obeying the normal rules that govern cell behaviour. Progesterone appears to have a natural regulating influence on the womb lining cells – it's the brake whereas oestrogen is the accelerator. In the presence of oestrogen but absence of progesterone some womb lining cells are overproduced and over time some eventually lose control and can become cancerous.

It was discovered that by adding progesterone-like drugs (there are several types and the general term for them is 'progestogen') to the oestrogen the problem of endometrial cancer was much reduced, although not eliminated. The usual name for HRT that uses both oestrogen and progestogen is 'combined HRT'.

The use of oestrogen on its own ('unopposed oestrogen') is not safe in women who still have their uterus, no matter when in relation to their menopause they start taking HRT. They need to take combined HRT. Conversely, women who have had their uterus removed and who are otherwise suitable to take HRT need only take oestrogen and can dispense with the progestogen.

Types of hormones in use

Combinations of natural and synthetic chemical processes today make the various hormones available. Some use soy or yams as source material, others extract the oestrogens from pregnant mares' urine and yet others use entirely artificial means to produce them. Drug company chemists have produced a range of oestrogens and progestogens not so much because they think they can do better than nature but rather to overcome practical problems associated with getting the hormones into the body where they can do their work. All medicines taken by mouth have to run the gauntlet of being digested by stomach acid and the enzymes of the intestines and they then face being turned into some other chemical by the body's own processing plant, the liver. To enable the hormones inside tablets to survive these hurdles intact, changes to their chemical nature are made, but the original hormone activity is still preserved.

The differences in the precise chemical nature of the oestrogens and progestogens used in the various types of HRT do not appear to be important as far as their ability to relieve the general symptoms of the menopause is concerned. They all do that very well. As far as bone protection is concerned, however, it is only the oestrogen content that is important.

The types of oestrogen and progestogen used in HRT are very similar to those used in the oral contraceptive pill. However, the strength of the oestrogen used in HRT is several times less than that used in the pill.

Forms of HRT available

Although there are dozens of individual brands of HRT available for a doctor to prescribe, they break down into a smaller number of categories:

LOCAL TREATMENTS

Oestrogen creams, tablets ('pessaries') or rings inserted high in the vagina which are impregnated with oestrogen that slowly leaks out, for the relief of vaginal symptoms such as dryness, irritation and pain on intercourse. These treatments do not deliver a sufficient amount of oestrogen to the rest of the body, so they are not suitable for the prevention of osteoporosis.

GENERAL TREATMENTS

Oral (tablets of oestrogen alone or along with progesterone in combined HRT preparations), patches and gels (which deliver the hormones through the skin), implants (small rods impregnated with hormone that are inserted under the skin and release oestrogen slowly over many months) and nasal sprays are the forms available. These can all provide sufficient doses of oestrogen to the whole body to be used for osteoporosis.

HRT and bone protection

The degree of protection from osteoporosis that HRT provides depends on how long the HRT is used. As soon as HRT is stopped, assuming that a woman taking it is already past the menopause, then the bones begin to lose strength as they would do naturally and it is not certain whether the rate of bone loss following cessation of HRT is quicker than the rate following the menopause. Until fairly recently a period of 10 years' treatment was often suggested as the optimum length of time for maximum bone protection, while minimising the risks of HRT. There has, however, been a shake-up of opinion over the use of HRT in postmenopausal women in the recent past.

Several large research studies were set up, principally in the USA and the UK, and reported their main results in 2002. The Women's Health Initiative Study (WHI) in particular has been the most influential in changing expert opinion. This was a large American study involving over 16,000 women who were post-menopausal and in the age range 50–79. It used a form of HRT that is not the same as that used in the UK. The trial was planned to last 8.5 years but was stopped early at 5.2 years because of an increase in the number of women on HRT who were developing breast cancer. Increases were also seen in coronary heart disease, stroke and vein thrombosis. However, there were reductions in hip fracture and colon cancer in those patients on HRT.

Use of HRT

HRT does not directly cause heart disease, strokes, breast cancer or vein thrombosis. These are all conditions that also occur in women who don't take HRT and there are many other factors that can increase a woman's risk that are unrelated to hormones, such as her family history, smoking history, blood pressure and cholesterol level to mention only a few. We don't know precisely why these risk factors matter, but the more that are present the more likely it is that the chain of events that leads to these health problems will be set in motion.

In summary, the use of HRT is not now recommended as first-line treatment for long-term prevention of osteoporosis in women over 50 years of age. It may still be an option for older women with a particularly high risk of osteoporosis, and an expert in osteoporosis should in any case advise such women on the various treatments and risks.

Expert advice in respect of younger women has, however, not changed. Women who experience an early menopause (under 45 years) should be offered HRT until they are 50 years old unless there are other reasons against doing so. In postmenopausal women between 45 and 50 the decision needs to be made on individual circumstances but would still tend to be in favour of using HRT at least for a few years.

The controversy surrounding HRT has perhaps cast a darker cloud over it than need be. HRT can give marked relief from many of the symptoms of the menopause and when used sensibly is still an appropriate treatment for a great many women. Many critics of HRT have maintained that it has tended to be over-prescribed and this may be true. Women at ordinary or low risk of osteoporosis should not now receive HRT for bone protection only, but those at high risk of osteoporosis should be expertly advised before deciding whether or not to take it.

Key Points

- Oestrogen-containing HRT slows the rate at which bone is lost in women following the menopause and may even reverse the process of osteoporosis, at least temporarily.
- The benefits of HRT on bone strength last only as long as the HRT is being taken.
- The use of HRT in postmenopausal women is now recommended only up to the age of about 55.
- HRT is still recommended for the majority of women who undergo an early menopause, especially those under 45.

Chapter 8

Prevention and Treatment of Osteoporosis: (c) Other Drug Treatments

Over the past decade several additional medicines have become available to protect against bone loss or to treat established osteoporosis. The two main ways in which this can be achieved are either by slowing down the rate of loss of bone (by blocking the activity of the osteoclast cells) or by speeding up the action of the bone-forming cells (osteoblasts).

Oestrogen stimulates the osteoblasts and the loss of this stimulation is why postmenopausal osteoporosis occurs, and why HRT is effective at slowing it down. The most commonly used non-HRT drugs for osteoporosis work instead on the osteoclasts, by slowing the rate at which these cells break down surrounding bone into its component materials – the process known as 'resorption'.

Bisphosphonates

'Bisphosphonate' is the chemical name for a group of drugs that can block the activity of osteoclasts. They work by becoming adsorbed on to the surface of the crystals that form the microscopic structure of bone and they thereby slow the rate at which these crystals can be dissolved by the osteoclasts. The bisphosphonates have become the most widely used drugs in osteoporosis management and there are three presently in common use (the brand names are listed in brackets):

1 Etidronate (Didronel PMO®)
2 Alendronate (Fosamax®)
3 Risedronate (Actonel®)

Etidronate was the first bisphosphonate and is still in widespread use, although it is now considered second choice to alendronate and risedronate. If etidronate is given continuously it blocks the addition of minerals to bone, which is the reverse of the desired effect. To get round this problem it is given in pulses of one tablet daily for 14 days and then a calcium tablet is taken daily for the next 76 days. Then the next 90-day treatment cycle starts again. After several years of treatment etidronate causes up to about 5 per cent increase in bone density in the lower part of the spine (lumbar area). Etidronate is marketed under the trade name of Didronel PMO®.

Alendronate and *risedronate* are newer bisphosphonates and are now the first choice in this group. Unlike etidronate they do not block bone mineralisation if given continuously, and they improve bone strength throughout the skeleton, not just within the spine.

These drugs can therefore be taken daily, but a convenient once-a-week form is available for both, which works just as well. Alendronate is marketed as Fosamax® or Fosamax Once Weekly® and risedronate as Actonel® or Actonel Once a Week®.

As with any drug taken by mouth and active within the body, the amount of drug absorbed by the digestive system has a very important bearing on how well the drug works. Unfortunately all of the bisphosphonates are very poorly absorbed – between 1 and 5 per cent only of the oral dose gets into the body. They therefore need to be taken on an empty stomach, which means, for example, in the morning 30 minutes before breakfast, or during the day in the middle of a four-hour fast. Occasionally they can cause irritation of the gullet (oesophagus) so they need to be washed down with plenty of water and taken while sitting or standing up.

The results of treatment with bisphosphonates are significant and have been demonstrated in several large research studies. Roughly speaking these drugs, given over a period of two to four years, halve the risk of subsequent fracture when given to post-menopausal women with a prior history of osteoporotic spinal fracture. Etidronate reduces spinal fracture risk but alendronate and risedronate also reduce the risk of fractures of non-spinal bones such as the hip.

The bisphosphonates can all be used to prevent or treat osteoporosis caused by prolonged steroid drug treatment. Etidronate and alendronate can be used in males with osteoporosis, whereas risedronate is licensed only for use in postmenopausal women.

Selective Estrogen Receptor Modulator (SERM)

This is a fairly new type of drug, of which raloxifene (Evista®) is presently the only one available. Raloxifene stimulates bone growth just as oestrogens do but has an anti-oestrogen effect on the uterus (womb) and on breast tissue. The latter effect is seen as desirable as it may reduce the tendency for long-term oestrogen-based HRT to increase the risk of developing breast cancer.

To a similar extent as HRT, raloxifene may increase the risk of developing blood clots in the veins and so it cannot be used by a woman with a past history of deep vein thrombosis (DVT). It is preferably used only in women who are five years past their menopause and would be an option for a woman between about 55 and 70 years of age. In research trials raloxifene, given with calcium and vitamin D supplements, has been shown to reduce the occurrence of spinal fractures by about a third, but it had no significant effect on hip or other non-spinal fractures.

Calcium and vitamin D supplements

The roles of calcium and vitamin D in osteoporosis were mentioned in chapter 2. The value of ensuring adequate intakes of these two basic nutrients is well illustrated in the case of elderly housebound women, including those who are in long-term care. Without selecting patients on the basis of DXA scans, the addition of calcium and vitamin D can reduce the occurrence of hip and other fractures by up to 35 per cent. The results of treating elderly men are less clear but are still likely to be beneficial. A number of proprietary and non-proprietary combination tablets (or sachets) containing calcium and vitamin D are available and are prescribable on the NHS. Taking these supplements at the standard dosage (usually one or two tablets or sachets daily) is perfectly safe, and does not have to be accompanied by blood tests to monitor calcium or vitamin D levels. If everyone over the age of 80 were encouraged to take this simple treatment the impact on fracture occurrence would be considerable.

Drugs used less often in osteoporosis

CALCITONIN

Calcitonin is a hormone naturally produced from the thyroid gland in the neck and which is involved in the control of calcium use. Calcitonin stops osteoclast cells from breaking down bone (resorption), hence its potential use in the treatment of osteoporosis. Calcitonin can also reduce the pain of a vertebral fracture, although it is not formally licensed for such use in the UK. It is available both as an injection and as a nasal spray. In the UK calcitonin would be prescribed only on the advice of a specialist in bone diseases.

TERIPARATIDE

This is a recently available genetically engineered compound derived from parathyroid hormone, which is another of the body's natural hormones involved in calcium control. It is available for use under specialist guidance for patients with severe osteoporosis and has to be given by daily injection for an 18-month course.

Drug combinations

One of the questions presently under investigation is whether the combination of HRT or raloxifene along with a bisphosphonate gives better results than using only one of these drugs (along with calcium and/or vitamin D supplements). Preliminary results suggest that there may be benefits in such combinations but as yet not enough is known to make any recommendations.

Strontium

Although not yet available as a treatment, strontium is one of those drugs showing promise in osteoporosis research. In one recent study strontium given over three years to a group of post-meno-pausal women with osteoporosis reduced the risk of spinal fracture by over 40 per cent.

National Institute for Clinical Excellence (NICE) guidance on osteoporosis drug treatment

NICE is a body set up by the government to provide doctors with advice on the effectiveness and use of drugs and other forms of treatment in a wide range of medical conditions. At the time of writing (May 2004) the final guidance from NICE on the management of osteoporosis is still awaited but draft guidance issued at the end of 2003 caused considerable concern among many experts and the support groups in osteoporosis and charities such as the National Osteoporosis Society.

Among the draft proposals from NICE was the recommendation that osteoporosis treatment should be limited to those people who had already suffered an osteoporotic fracture. This effectively would have meant closing the door on using medicines to prevent osteoporotic fractures happening in the first place, and caused much protest. Another proposal that caused concern was a recommendation to treat women over 65 with a 'fragility fracture' without doing DXA scanning first. Experts pointed out that osteoporosis is not the only cause of fractures and putting a woman on to long-term treatment without confirming the diagnosis would not be sensible in many cases.

Among several other proposals that were widely criticised, NICE originally ruled out raloxifene as a treatment for osteoporosis. The updated draft guidance (May 2004) has reinstated raloxifene as a second-line treatment option for women who cannot take or are otherwise unsuitable for bisphosphonates. The final NICE guidance on osteoporosis treatment is expected by October 2004.

At first sight it may appear that NICE guidance is at variance with expert opinion, but some caution is required before being too sure. NICE does indeed have many critics but the organisation does go to great lengths to assess information objectively and to come up with fair and balanced views. Sometimes their opinions challenge the status quo, and so generate some friction. It is true nonetheless that the majority of studies into the effectiveness of the drugs used in osteoporosis have been done on patients who already have had at least one osteoporotic fracture. We know that bisphosphonates have a large impact on this group of people, and it is natural that we should wish to close the stable door before the horse has bolted by trying to prevent first fractures occurring – in other words by giving these drugs for 'primary prevention'. What the NICE guidance has reflected is that the amount of evidence supporting the use of drugs to prevent osteoporosis, at least in people below 60 years of age, is limited. It seems, on the basis of how we think the drugs work, that it would be a good idea to give these drugs to people at risk but we still have a great deal of work to do before we can be sure when is a good time to start treatment and how long we should take the drugs in order to get the most benefit.

The evidence for people over 60 and for those who have had an osteoporotic fracture is much more robust. Essentially, we know that these are the groups of people for whom bisphosphonates and to a lesser extent the other drugs have a strong place. Osteoporosis, as with so much of modern medicine, is not a field of knowledge that is all tidily sorted out. Our understanding of the condition and how to tackle it is still basic and in need of more research. Undoubtedly what we think now is best practice will be changed in a few years when more information is available. The best that we can presently manage is to consider targeting treatment at the highest risk groups of people, as noted earlier in this book. If we do this well we will make a huge impact on the disability caused by osteoporosis. As time goes by we will know better how to prevent osteoporosis occurring, but even as present knowledge stands we can be sure that it is lifestyle factors such as diet and exercise that have the greatest impact on this condition, not drug treatment.

Before rounding off the book with some advice on other measures to deal with osteoporosis, we need to take a bit of space to cover the male of the species, and how the condition affects him too.

Key Points

- The bisphosphonates are drugs that can block the activity of osteoclasts, thereby slowing the rate at which bone is broken down.
- Alendronate and risedronate are the preferred bisphosphonate drugs in current use.
- Raloxifene (Evista) is an alternative drug for osteoporosis that can be used in women only.
- Taking a simple supplement of calcium and vitamin D can significantly reduce the likelihood of fragility fracture in elderly women, and probably also in elderly men.
- Calcitonin and teriparatide are drugs used in people with more severe osteoporosis who cannot tolerate or fail to improve with other medications, or who are recommended them by an osteoporosis specialist.

Chapter 9

Osteoporosis and Men

Awareness that osteoporosis also affects men is increasing but it is still low compared to osteoporosis in women, including among health professionals. However, the same sorts of signs should raise the suspicion of osteoporosis in a man as in a woman. For example, a man who has had a fracture after relatively little trauma, or who shows signs of height loss, should be investigated for osteoporosis. Men can benefit from all of the general and some of the more specific osteoporosis treatments that apply to women.

In women the cessation of periods is an obvious outward sign that the menopause has occurred. In men there is no obvious physical sign that is the male equivalent of periods stopping. Whether the 'male menopause' exists at all is a controversial area and detailed coverage of the pros and cons of such a concept are beyond the scope of this book. However, the under-recognition of male osteoporosis can only be improved if we get better at recognising the signs and symptoms that may accompany it, so a brief overview is well justified.

Does the 'male menopause' exist?

There is a difficulty with defining the male menopause because measuring testosterone levels is far from straightforward and what might be a normal level in one man may represent a deficiency in another. Put another way, the problem with defining a male menopause is in deciding when natural aging has merged into something more pervasive and which merits treatment.

MALE AGING

The testes are the main sites of production of the male sex hormones, predominant among which is testosterone. Although men can retain the ability to produce active sperm in the testes throughout their lives the output of testosterone declines with age. Men undoubtedly experience symptoms caused by the drop in sex hormones but individuals are affected differently. Some men experience very few symptoms, whereas others are completely disabled by them. Although this fall in sex hormone production is a natural process and not a disease, it still merits recognition and, in some men, treatment. Testosterone is not the only hormone that undergoes changes in production in an older man but the significance of the other hormones is even less clear.

The mental and physical changes that can occur in men are much more subtle in onset, may take many years or even decades to become apparent and can easily be missed. As such, the term 'male menopause', or 'andropause', is probably not accurate. Instead, experts prefer to talk about 'partial androgen deficiency of the ageing male' (PADAM). ('Androgen' is the general term for the 'male hormones', including testosterone.)

THE SYMPTOMS OF ANDROGEN DEFICIENCY

The symptoms of PADAM are numerous and are shared with many other medical conditions including depression, so it is not an easy condition to diagnose. They include hot flushes, sweating, poor sleep, irritability, tiredness, nervousness, lack of motivation, difficulty with short-term memory, depression, diminished muscle strength, decreased interest in or desire for sex and many more. Physical features can include diminished muscle mass, loss of body hair and 'abdominal obesity', which is where excess weight is put on mostly around the tummy area.

Several other effects on body chemistry and metabolism occur, such as a rise in the type of blood cholesterol that increases the risk of developing coronary artery disease, an increase in total body fat (because of a fall in the proportion of body weight that is muscle rather than through weight gain), and osteoporosis. Many of these symptoms, signs and metabolic consequences can be corrected by androgen replacement therapy.

DIAGNOSING AND TREATING ANDROGEN DEFICIENCY

As with the female menopause, no definitive test for PADAM exists. Low blood levels of testosterone alone are insufficient to make the diagnosis. The combination of several different suggestive symptoms and physical signs, together with low blood levels of testosterone, should raise suspicion that PADAM is present. Because of the difficulties, men suspected of having PADAM should see an expert with a special interest in this problem.

Treatment also raises many difficulties, not least because many doctors do not believe that PADAM exists and will not offer treatment. Testosterone treatment may stimulate the growth of the prostate gland or a pre-existing cancer of the prostate gland, which is an increasingly common type of cancer, especially in older men. Monitoring of blood cholesterol is required as it may become undesirably high. Having said that, the appropriate use of testosterone replacement in older men severely affected by androgen deficiency can considerably improve their quality of life.

Osteoporosis, men and 'HRT'

Testosterone replacement is the male equivalent of oestrogen replacement in women – it's a man's 'HRT'. Theoretically one of the benefits of giving testosterone to a man who has PADAM should be that osteoporosis is halted or even improved, as occurs in women on oestrogen replacement. Unfortunately this area of treatment lacks research. Testosterone replacement has been shown to improve bone mineral density but has not yet been shown to have a positive effect upon a man's long-term risk of getting a bone fracture, which is really what matters most.

Men who have normal levels of testosterone (bearing in mind how difficult that is to define) do not show improvements in bone mineral density when given testosterone supplements, so it is important to target testosterone treatment only to those men who need it.

The present position concerning osteoporosis and testosterone replacement in men is therefore unclear and it is not possible to make generalisations. There are men who need and are helped by testosterone treatment, and it is likely that such treatment also improves bone strength. A good deal more research is needed before one can say much more than that.

Treatment of male osteoporosis

BISPHOSPHONATES

Fewer studies have been done on the results of treating men with bisphosphonates than on women, although in theory they should work equally well. Alendronate (Fosamax®), combined with calcium and vitamin D supplements, has been shown to increase bone mineral density and reduce the rate of bone fracture in men with established osteoporosis. Only the once-daily form of Fosamax® is presently licensed in the UK for use in men, although the once-a-week form is likely to be as effective. Etidronate (Didronel PMO®) may also be used in men.

CALCIUM AND VITAMIN D SUPPLEMENTS

Equally, although the value of calcium and vitamin D in postmenopausal women is well established, it is not clear whether these supplements are as effective in men. Bearing in mind that the treatment is safe and that the disability from osteoporotic fracture is sometimes worse in men, it is reasonable to offer these supplements at least to older men with impaired mobility or those who are in long-term residential care.

Key Points

- An unknown percentage of older men suffer from a lack of testosterone (androgen) that could be helped by testosterone replacement.
- The diagnosis of androgen deficiency is difficult and should be done by a specialist.
- Testosterone replacement would be likely to benefit some men with osteoporosis but more research is needed to clarify which men should be targeted.
- Bisphosphonates can be used to treat osteoporosis in men.

Chapter 10

Other Points

Steroid drugs and osteoporosis

Medical treatment with steroid drugs is the commonest reason for so called 'secondary' osteoporosis, i.e. osteoporosis caused by something else.

Steroid drugs can have dramatic positive benefits in a great many medical conditions, and may well be life saving in, for example, severe asthma. For as long as we've known how useful they are we have, however, also realised that they have their downside. If taken at high enough dose for several weeks or more then a range of side effects start to appear, such as retention of body fluid, weight gain, puffy face and ankles, raised blood pressure, thinning and easy bruising of the skin, a tendency to diabetes and a weakening of the bones, among others.

Doctors therefore try to use the shortest possible course of steroids at the smallest dose that achieves the desired effect, but often it is impossible to avoid the need for longer-term use of steroids, which is when some anticipation of the effects this may have on bone strength becomes necessary.

It is important to re-emphasise that the dose of steroids present in treatments such as asthma inhalers is not sufficient to cause osteoporosis and so need not cause any worry in that regard. The over-use of very potent steroid creams by people with severe eczema can lead to significant absorption of steroid into the body but the vast majority of people who use steroid creams at ordinary dosages and strengths should also have no need to be concerned. If you do have such concerns then you should discuss them with your GP.

The type of steroid treatment that we need to take care with is the oral form, such as prednisolone tablets, and 'long-term' as far as the bones are concerned means three months or longer.

PEOPLE 65 YEARS OR OVER

Older people are at the most risk from steroid-induced osteoporosis and the majority will be best served by taking one of the bisphosphonate drugs (alendronate, risedronate, etidronate) from the start of the steroid treatment, if it is known in advance that the steroids will need to be taken for a while. In some medical conditions it only becomes clear after some time that the steroids will need to be continued for long enough to matter, so the bisphosphonate can start then. Calcium and vitamin D supplements should also be considered and most of the time it will be a good idea to take these too.

PEOPLE UNDER 65 YEARS OLD

It is a bit more complex to decide on when to use 'bone-protection' on younger people. Current guidelines (appendix A) define two sub groups:

1. Those with no history of a previous osteoporotic fracture

Ideally these people should have a bone mineral density scan. If it shows normal BMD with a T score above 0 then unless very high doses of steroid are likely to be used it will be enough for them to keep up a good intake of calcium-rich foods in their diet and take regular exercise. Of course this may be more difficult depending on the medical condition for which they need steroids in the first place, so it is only general advice and has to be tailored to the individual.

For those in this group whose BMD is between 0 and –1.5 a closer eye is needed. They should use the general measures of diet and exercise, of course, but will need a repeat bone mineral density scan in one to three years if the steroids are to continue this long.

Those with a BMD of –1.5 or lower need to start bone-protecting treatment right away, as for the over 65 group.

2. Those with a previous history of osteoporotic fracture, or who develop one during their steroid treatment

People in this group should be managed as for the over 65 group, and need to start bone-protecting treatment right away.

Fall risk

If you remember back to chapter 1, we mentioned that the outcome for anyone with osteoporosis really depended on the interplay of three factors: bone strength, risk of falling and the nature of the injury.

Fall risk can depend on so many other factors that it really is a topic that needs a separate book. Obvious home hazards such as loose carpets or clutter that can cause someone to trip may be easily dealt with, but other issues such as a person's sight, hearing, balance, mobility, drug therapy and more all come into play. You can get help with fall risk, for yourself or for a relative or friend, by simply asking for it via your primary care team (GP, Practice Nurse, Health Visitor) or through the local Social Services department. Physiotherapists and Occupational Therapists tend to be the professional groups most involved in this sort of care and they much prefer prevention to treatment.

Hip protectors

Fractures of the hip (femur) are the biggest single group of osteoporotic fractures causing the largest amount of disability. Hip protectors are shock-absorbing pads that come as a sort of girdle with padding at the sides. Should someone fall they help to spread the impact over a large area of the upper leg, which can help reduce the chance of fracture occurring. Although hip protectors can provide a worthwhile degree of extra protection they are clearly only a partial solution. It is also self-evident that they do not work unless they are worn! It can be difficult for someone always to remember to put it on, or wish to keep it on.

Vertegroplasty

Tiny fractures of the spine in osteoporosis can accumulate over time and lead to the progressive forward stoop mentioned earlier. Often this type of spinal fracturing is not painful. Osteoporosis may, however, also result in a more abrupt and significant spinal fracture that can be very painful indeed. Painkillers are the first line of treatment and may need to be of high strength to be effective.

The pain from a collapsed vertera may last for a considerable length of time.

Vertebroplasty is a technique in which acrylic bone cement is injected into the middle of the collapsed vertebra via a hypodermic needle. Despite sounding complex, this can be done under local anaesthetic and X-ray pictures are taken to guide the needle accurately. When the cement hardens it is very strong and it prevents movement of the bone gragments. This can be very effective at reducing the pain. Vertebroplasty, when carried out by skilled personnel, appears very safe but it is not suitable for all patients, nor is it widely available as a treatment in the UK.

Vertebroplasty is a treatment for pain only. It does not do anything for the deformity or loss of height that can occur with a spinal fracture. A development of the technique is first to insert a balloon into the space occupied by the fractured vertebra and then to inflate it under pressure to expand the space back to as near normal as possible. This corrects the forward collapse and height loss. The balloon is then withdrawn and the cavity it has caused is filled with bone cement to stabilise it. This technique, called kyphoplasty, is even less available in the UK than vertebroplasty.

Both techniques have their supporters and their critics. The former cite patients whose pain has successfully been relieved whereas the latter point out that most bone fractures heal eventually without treatment and that strengthening one vertebra may case another fracture to occur higher up the spine. All one can say here is that the treatments are available but expert guidance is needed on their suitability for any individual.

Conclusions

Osteoporosis is ideally a condition that should be prevented from occurring, but that is an unrealistic aim given our present state of knowledge and ability to influence it. It should, however, be obvious from the preceding chapters that healthy bones at least partially reflect healthy living.

Taking regular exercise is the single most important action anyone can take to improve the strength of their bones. Exercise also greatly reduces the risk of heart disease, high blood pressure and diabetes and it has positive effects on mental well-being too. The sort of exercise that is beneficial is weight bearing, such as walking or aerobics, depending on whether you have already developed osteoporosis or are trying to prevent yourself from doing so. You can get advice on what to do from your local physiotherapy department – so make good use of it!

Stopping smoking should be a priority for anyone interested in enjoying a longer life as well as keeping away from orthopaedic wards, and alcohol consumption should be kept within safe limits.

A good calcium intake is essential throughout life for healthy bones and there is good evidence that the adequacy of a child's diet at least partially determines their osteoporosis risk in adulthood. There is more information in appendix D about high-calcium foods. Taking a supplement of calcium along with vitamin D may help frail elderly people with poor mobility.

Everyone can use these general measures, whether or not they ultimately are shown to have osteoporosis. Checking through the list of high risk factors in chapter 4 will help you to decide if osteoporosis is something you might be prone to getting, if it has not already occurred. Take this information to your GP and discuss it if you think you might be at increased risk, or are just looking for reassurance that all is well.

As far as bone density scanning is concerned the situation is not ideal. Waiting times for such tests around the country vary enormously, from weeks in some areas to over a year in others. The current advice from the National Institute for Clinical Excellence is confusing and essentially means that the majority of women will need a bone density scan result before the GP can decide on treatment. Hopefully the finalised guidelines from NICE, due to be issued in late 2004, will be clear and practical.

It is still fairly early days in our understanding of this important condition, which is set to become even more common as our population gets older, and if present trends continue, to be more sedentary and less fit in the true sense. We do not yet have cures but we do have safe treatments that can make a real difference, and many more people could benefit from such treatment than presently receive it.

We all need to be more 'bone aware', doctors included, as an important part of keeping ourselves fit and healthy into our old age.

Appendix A

References and Contacts

References

GENERAL

- British Medical Journal collected resources on osteoporosis: http://bmj.bmjjournals.com/cgi/collection/osteoporosis
- New England Journal of Medicine collected resources: http://content.nejm.org/collections (look under Bone disease)
- National Institute for Clinical Excellence: www.nice.org.uk (osteoporosis guidelines listed in 'Technology Appraisals')
- Scottish Intercollegiate Guidelines Network: www.sign.ac.uk; 'Guideline 71: Management of Osteoporosis', June 2003: www.sign.ac.uk/guidelines/fulltext/71/index.html
- National Osteoporosis Society, 'A Primary Care Strategy for Osteoporosis and Falls': www.nos.org.uk/PDF/PCGDoc2002.pdf

(this is a link to the document from within the National Osteoporosis Society's website)
- Fogelman, I., 'Screening for osteoporosis' (British Medical Journal, 1999; 319:1148–49); http://bmj.bmjjournals.com/cgi/content/full/319/7218/1148

MENOPAUSE AND HRT
- Cranney, A., 'Treatment of postmenopausal osteoporosis' (British Medical Journal, 2003; 327: 355–56); http://bmj.bmjjournals.com/cgi/content/full/327/7411/355
- McPherson, K., 'Where are we now with hormone replacement therapy?' (British Medical Journal, 2004; 328: 357–58); http://bmj.bmjjournals.com/cgi/content/full/328/7436/357
- Bruyere, O., et al., 'Fracture prevention in postmenopausal women' (Clinical Evidence, 2003; 10: 1304–22); www.clinical evidence.com/ceweb/conditions/index.jsp or link from website for National Electronic Library for Health: www.nelh.nhs.uk

OSTEOPOROSIS IN MEN
- Orwoll, E., et al., 'Alendronate for the treatment of men' (New England Journal of Medicine, 2000; 343: 604–10); http://content.nejm.org/cgi/content/abstract/343/9/604

OTHER TOPICS
- Hodson, J., and Marsh, J., 'Quantitative ultrasound and risk factor enquiry as predictors of postmenopausal osteoporosis: comparative study in primary care' (British Medical Journal, 2003; 326: 1250–51); http://bmj.bmjjournals.com/cgi/content/full/326/7401/1250
- Tylavsky, F.A., et al., 'Fruit and vegetable intakes are an independent predictor of bone size in early pubertal children'

(American Journal of Clinical Nutrition, 2004; 79(2): 311–17); http://www.ajcn.org/cgi/content/abstract/79/2/311
- Woolf, A., and Åkesson, K., 'Preventing fractures in elderly people' (British Medical Journal, 2003; 327: 89–95); http://bmj.bmjjournals.com/cgi/content/full/327/7406/89
- The Chartered Society of Physiotherapy: 'Physiotherapy Guidelines for the Management of Osteoporosis' (1999); can be downloaded from: http://admin.csp.org.uk/admin2/uploads/-38c9a362-ed71ce5fa5-7ff5/OSTEOgl.pdf

Contacts

NATIONAL OSTEOPOROSIS SOCIETY
The National Osteoporosis Society is the only national charity dedicated to improving the diagnosis, prevention and treatment of the condition.

National Osteoporosis Society
Camerton
Bath BA2 0PJ
Tel: 01761 471771 (for general enquiries)
Helpline: 0845 4500230 (for medical queries)
Fax: 01761 471104
Email: info@nos.org.uk
Website: www.nos.org.uk

INTERNATIONAL OSTEOPOROSIS FOUNDATION
Website: www.osteofound.org

Appendix B

Drugs

The following information contains selected details of some of the medications used in treating osteoporosis. Where more than one product is available in a particular group only one is described as an example. Full details are included in the manufacturer's data sheets and can also be viewed within the medicines section of the NetDoctor web site http://www.netdoctor.co.uk/medicines/

The information is accurate at the time of writing but new information on medicines appears regularly. A health professional should always be consulted concerning the prescription and use of medicines.

Medicines and their possible side effects can affect individual people in different ways. The following lists some of the side effects that are known to be associated with these medicines. Side effects other than those listed may exist.

Alendronate

HOW DOES IT WORK?

This medicine contains the active ingredient alendronate sodium, which is a type of medicine called a bisphosphonate. These agents are used in a variety of metabolic bone disorders. Bisphosphonates work by binding very tightly to bone, preventing the removal of calcium from the bone cells. This decreases breakdown and turnover of bone in the body and the increased calcium content leads to stronger bones.

In osteoporosis, bone turnover is increased, causing the bones to become weak and prone to breaking. This medicine slows down the process of bone breakdown, so keeping bones stronger and helping to prevent fractures. It is used to treat osteoporosis and prevent fractures in people with the disease, and also to prevent bone loss in people at risk of developing osteoporosis.

CAUTIONS

Food, drinks (except plain water) and certain other medicines such as calcium supplements and antacids taken by mouth may interfere with the absorption of this medicine from the gut. For this reason you should wait at least 30 minutes after taking alendronate before taking any other medicines by mouth.

You should stop taking this medicine and seek medical attention if you experience difficulty or pain on swallowing, new or worsening heartburn, or pain behind the breastbone.

It is very important that the dosing instructions for this medicine are followed completely. This is because the medicine can cause irritation and ulceration of the gullet (oesophagus). Following the instructions correctly minimises this risk. The tablets must be swallowed whole with a glass of plain water (at least 200ml, not mineral water), and not sucked or chewed. You should sit or stand for at least 30 minutes after taking the tablet to aid its movement into the stomach. For this reason don't take the tablet before getting up in the morning or less than 30 minutes before going to bed at night.

MAIN SIDE EFFECTS
- Headache
- Rash
- Excess gas in the stomach and intestines (flatulence)
- Disturbances of the gut such as diarrhoea, constipation, nausea, vomiting or abdominal pain
- Swelling of abdomen
- Indigestion
- Low blood calcium level
- Pain in muscles or bones
- Flushing of the skin
- Inflammation or ulceration of the gullet
- Difficulty or pain when swallowing
- Acid regurgitation
- Light-sensitive skin reactions
- Inflammation of the front parts of the eye (uveitis)

BRAND NAMES
Fosamax®, Fosamax Once Weekly®

Raloxifene

HOW DOES IT WORK?
This medicine contains the active ingredient raloxifene hydrochloride, which is a type of medicine called a selective oestrogen receptor modulator (SERM).

Oestrogen, the main female hormone, has many actions throughout the body. Bone tissue, cholesterol metabolism, breast tissue and uterine tissue are all affected by this hormone. At the menopause, blood levels of oestrogen start to decrease and this affects the tissues that are normally responsive to oestrogen.

In terms of bone tissue, declining levels of oestrogen result in an increase in bone breakdown, which can lead to a loss of bone density. Bone loss is particularly rapid for the first ten years after the menopause and it may lead to the development of osteoporosis.

Raloxifene is used to both prevent and treat osteoporosis in postmenopausal women. It works by acting on oestrogen receptors in the bone tissue, where it mimics the natural effects of oestrogen. This gradually reverses the excessive breakdown of bone that happens at menopause and causes an increase in bone mineral density, making bones stronger. Raloxifene has been shown to significantly reduce the risk of spinal fractures, but not hip fractures.

Raloxifene selectively mimics the effects of oestrogen on bone tissue, but does not affect breast tissue or uterine tissue. This means that long-term use does not carry the increased risk of cancer of the lining of the womb (endometrial cancer) or breast cancer that is associated with long-term use of oestrogen-based hormone replacement therapy (HRT). However, raloxifene is associated with an increased risk of developing blood clots in the veins. This risk is similar to that associated with HRT.

Due to its selective activity, raloxifene is not effective at relieving other symptoms of oestrogen deficiency that occur during the menopause, for example hot flushes.

MAIN SIDE EFFECTS
- Headache
- Rash
- Abdominal pain

- Swelling of the legs and ankles due to excess fluid retention
- Indigestion
- Nausea and vomiting
- Leg cramps
- Hot flushes
- Migraine
- Increased risk of abnormal blood clots within the blood vessels
- Rise in blood pressure
- Decreased numbers of platelets in the blood

HOW CAN THIS MEDICINE AFFECT OTHER MEDICINES?

Raloxifene has not been studied in combination with medicines used to treat breast cancer, and it is not known what effect it might have on these medicines. For this reason, women with breast cancer should only take raloxifene after their breast cancer treatment has been completed.

The manufacturer of this medicine has not studied the effect of taking this medicine in combination with medicines that contain oestrogen, e.g. HRT. For this reason they recommend that it is not taken with oestrogen-containing medicines.

This medicine may reduce the blood-thinning effect of anticoagulant medicines such as warfarin. People taking an anticoagulant should have their blood clotting time checked after starting treatment with this medicine; any effect on blood clotting time may develop over several weeks.

BRAND NAME
Evista®

Calcium and vitamin D supplement – Example product: Adcal D3

HOW DOES IT WORK?

This medicine contains two active ingredients, calcium carbonate, which is a calcium salt used mainly to supplement calcium in the diet, and cholecalciferol, otherwise known as vitamin D3.

Calcium is needed for the formation of strong bones and healthy teeth and is involved in helping the blood to clot. It is also required to transmit nerve signals and help muscles work. Usually, calcium requirements are met from the diet. However, there are times when the amount of calcium required is increased, such as during pregnancy, when breastfeeding or with advancing age. When there is insufficient calcium in the diet to meet the body's needs, supplements are needed, otherwise calcium deficiency can occur.

Calcium supplements are useful in osteoporosis; a calcium intake that is twice the recommended daily allowance (RDA) slows the rate of bone loss and reduces the risk of fractures.

Cholecalciferol, also known as vitamin D3, is normally obtained primarily from sunlight acting on the skin. It is also consumed in the diet in oily fish and milk products. Vitamin D deficiency develops when there is inadequate exposure to sunlight, such as in elderly people with reduced mobility or who are housebound, or when there is a lack of the vitamin in the diet. Vitamin D is needed for calcium to be absorbed from the gut, and deficiency can lead to low calcium levels and subsequent weakening of bones. This is known as osteomalacia. Vitamin D supplements correct vitamin D deficiency and improve calcium absorption from the gut.

Calcium and vitamin D supplements are used to treat osteomalacia and osteoporosis. By increasing vitamin D and calcium in the body they help strengthen the bones. They are also used to supplement the diet during pregnancy, when there are increased requirements for these nutrients. Calcium and vitamin D supplements are also given to prevent and treat dietary deficiency, for example in the housebound elderly.

CAUTIONS
People with mild to moderate kidney failure, raised levels of calcium in the urine or a history of kidney stones may need the levels of calcium in their blood and urine to be regularly monitored while taking this medicine. Calcium-containing medicines can reduce the absorption of other drugs such as antibiotics, bisphosphonates, iron-containing preparations and thyroxine, and may interact with other medicines. Ask your pharmacist for advice on taking other medications with this one.

MAIN SIDE EFFECTS
- Constipation
- Diarrhoea
- Pain in the stomach and abdominal area
- Excess gas in the stomach and intestines (flatulence)
- Nausea
- Skin rashes
- High blood calcium level
- High calcium levels in the urine

OTHER MEDICINES CONTAINING THE SAME ACTIVE INGREDIENTS
Calcichew D3, Calcichew D3 Forte

Teriparatide

HOW DOES IT WORK?

This medicine contains the active ingredient teriparatide, which is a type of medicine called a bone formation agent. Teriparatide is a synthetic version of the human parathyroid hormone, produced by the parathyroid glands. This hormone is involved in the metabolism of calcium and phosphorus. Teriparatide mimics the effects of the natural human hormone and is used to increase bone formation.

Teriparatide is used to treat osteoporosis in postmenopausal women and works by increasing the action of the bone-forming cells, the osteoblasts. Teriparatide also increases the absorption of calcium from the intestine into the blood and the re-absorption of calcium from the kidneys into the blood. Teriparatide has been shown to significantly reduce the risk of spinal factures, but not hip fractures, in postmenopausal women. It is given as a daily injection under the skin of the thigh or abdomen, using an injection pen similar to those used by people with diabetes for injecting insulin.

MAIN SIDE EFFECTS

- Headache
- Depression
- Muscle cramps
- Fatigue
- Weight gain
- Low blood pressure
- Balance problems involving the inner ear (vertigo)
- Awareness of your heartbeat (palpitations)
- Dizziness
- Nausea and vomiting
- Low red blood cell count (anaemia)
- Difficulty in breathing

- Redness around injection site
- Weakness or loss of strength
- Chest pain
- Increased production of urine
- Increased sweating
- Raised cholesterol levels
- Limb pain
- Sciatica
- Reflux of stomach acid into the gullet (gastro-oesophageal reflux)

BRAND NAME
Forsteo®

Hormone Replacement Therapy

There are many available brands of hormone replacement therapy, containing oestrogen alone or oestrogen combined with a progesterone-like drug ('progestogen'). From the point of view of osteoporosis it is only the oestrogen content that is active, but women who still have their uterus need to take the type of HRT that also contains a progestogen ('combined' HRT). The potential side effects of all the various types of HRT are very similar. The following information is generally applicable.

Combined HRT contains forms of the naturally occurring female sex hormones, oestrogen and progesterone. In women with an intact womb, oestrogen stimulates the growth of the womb lining (endometrium). This can lead to endometrial cancer if the growth is 'unopposed' by the effect of a progestogen. If a woman has had her womb surgically removed (a hysterectomy), endometrial cancer is not a risk and progesterone is not necessary as part of HRT.

There are two main types of HRT. One type gives a continuous daily dose of both hormones, which normally results in the stopping of menstrual periods. This type, called continuous HRT, is recommended for women who are at least 12 months after their last natural menstrual bleed.

The other type of HRT uses the concept of 'cycle therapy'. In cycle (also called 'sequential') therapy the progesterone component is added for 10 to 14 days at the end of the cycle. This mimics the fluctuating levels of oestrogen and progesterone that occur in the natural menstrual cycle and results in the womb lining being shed as a menstrual period at the end of each month. Sequential combined HRT is usually used in women who have not yet ceased menstruation but who are otherwise deemed to need HRT.

MAIN SIDE EFFECTS

Women taking HRT appear to have a small increase in the risk of being diagnosed with breast cancer, compared with women who do not take HRT. However, this risk must be weighed against the benefits of taking HRT, such as prevention of osteoporosis. Women on HRT are advised to have regular breast examinations and mammograms, and to practise breast self-examination.

Women taking HRT have a slight increase in the risk of abnormal blood clot formation (deep vein thrombosis and pulmonary embolism) compared with women not taking HRT. All women, but particularly those with a personal or family history of thrombosis or other risk factors (e.g. severe varicose veins, obesity, recent surgery, immobility), should carefully discuss the risks and benefits of HRT with their doctor.

OTHER POSSIBLE SIDE EFFECTS
- Headache
- Dizziness or loss of balance
- Fatigue

- Awareness of the heartbeat (palpitations)
- Excessive fluid retention in the body tissues, resulting in swelling (oedema)
- Nosebleeds
- Vaginal discharge
- Hair loss
- High blood pressure
- Skin reactions such as rash and itch
- Depressed mood
- Changes in sex drive
- Gut disturbances such as heartburn, nausea, vomiting, bloating, wind and stomach pain
- Build-up of bile (biliary stasis)
- Breast tenderness/swelling/pain

Appendix C

Simple Exercise Regime in Osteoporosis

(These exercises are provided courtesy of Glasgow Royal Infirmary Physiotherapy Department.)

Regular weight bearing exercise, that is exercise in which you are supporting your own body weight, improves bone density in everyone and is an especially important part of the prevention and treatment of osteoporosis. Exercise can also improve posture, balance, mood and general health and can help reduce pain from many different causes, including arthritis.

The advice on the next few pages is necessarily general but you can get specific advice for yourself from your local physiotherapist. A referral from your GP is normally required to access the physiotherapy service.

There are four types of exercise that you should do at home and these are detailed below in the home exercise programme. First, some general points about them:

Stretching and flexibility

Flexibility is an important part of being fit and active. Try to stretch regularly at home and always stretch after you have warmed up. Remember to hold the muscle stretches gently, for about 30 seconds. Do not bounce. Stretching can also improve your posture, which is very important in osteoporosis.

Muscle strengthening

Stronger muscles help reduce pain, support your bones and joints and make it less likely for you to fall. When doing the strengthening exercises you should be working hard. Aim to build up to doing three sets of 12 repetitions of each exercise.

Balance

Balance is something we take for granted, until we lose it. Like everything else, balance takes practice to improve. Dancing and exercise to music and Tai Chi are other good ways to improve balance.

General fitness

To improve your fitness it is very important that you start slowly and build up gradually. Start by setting aside five or ten minutes, gradually increasing to 20 minutes of continuous exercise, three times a week. During exercise you should be slightly out of breath, but still able to talk. If you can't manage 20 minutes in one go, remember that every little bit helps. Choose a type of exercise that you enjoy. Before starting your workout you should warm up a little first, then stretch.

WEIGHT BEARING EXERCISES INCLUDE:

- Brisk walking
- Stair climbing
- Low impact aerobics
- Aqua aerobics

Swimming and cycling are non weight bearing exercises and therefore they do not improve bone density. However, they do improve fitness, muscle strength, flexibility and general health so they are good to do. Just ensure that you are also doing weight bearing exercises too.

When osteoporosis is present

Higher impact and more strenuous weight bearing exercises are appropriate for people who do not have osteoporosis and who are fit enough in general to undertake them. Such exercise helps prevent osteoporosis occurring. However, those people who have already developed osteoporosis need to take some care in the type of exercise they do. Your physiotherapist can guide you more precisely, but in general, if you have osteoporosis then you should avoid:

- Running or jogging
- Skipping
- High impact aerobics
- Jumping and hopping
- Repeated forward bending
- Fast twisting movements

Tips for exercising

Become more active in daily life. Walk to work or get off the bus one stop early and walk the rest of the way. Take the stairs instead of the lift. These changes will make a difference and you will be surprised how quickly your body will respond.

Find an activity that suits you. There is no point in forcing yourself to do something that you do not enjoy, but if you enjoy the activity then you will be more likely to keep it going in the long term. Try something new from time to time so you don't get bored. If you are taking up exercise for the first time or have any doubts about your suitability for doing so then ask your GP for advice.

REMEMBER
- Always work within your limits.
- Stop if an exercise causes pain or exacerbates any discomfort you already have.
- Make sure every exercise is controlled.
- If you become tired try slowing down instead of stopping.

Home exercise programme

The following exercises can be done at home any time you want. Although some of the exercises may be easy to you, it is important that you do them regularly to maintain your flexibility, strength and balance. You don't have to do all the exercises at once or all in the same day. For example, you could do half one day and the other half the next day. Or some in the morning and the rest in the afternoon. Try doing them with your favourite music playing.

The exercises are divided into three sections:

1. Flexibility
2. Strength
3. Balance

1. FLEXIBILITY

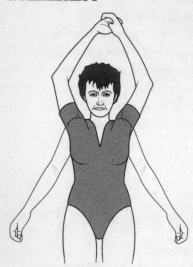

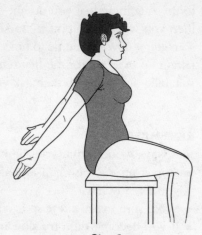

Step 1
Stand with hands clasped in front of you. Keeping arms straight, lift them forward and above your head. Separate your hands and bring them sideways to the starting position. Repeat five times.

Step 2
Sit with your back straight and feet on the floor. Pull your shoulder blades together while turning your thumbs and hands outwards, keeping your body straight. Hold for 20 seconds. Repeat three times.

Step 3
Sit straight backed. Pull your chin in, keeping your neck and back straight (not tipping your head forward), like making a double chin. Hold the end position and feel the stretching in the top part of your neck. Hold for 20 seconds. Repeat three times.

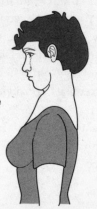

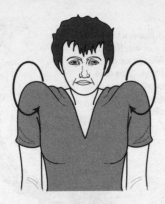

Step 4
Sit or stand. Circle your shoulders
backwards. Repeat five times.

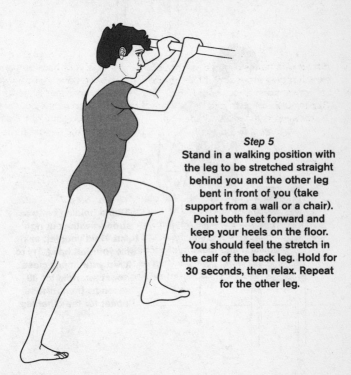

Step 5
Stand in a walking position with
the leg to be stretched straight
behind you and the other leg
bent in front of you (take
support from a wall or a chair).
Point both feet forward and
keep your heels on the floor.
You should feel the stretch in
the calf of the back leg. Hold for
30 seconds, then relax. Repeat
for the other leg.

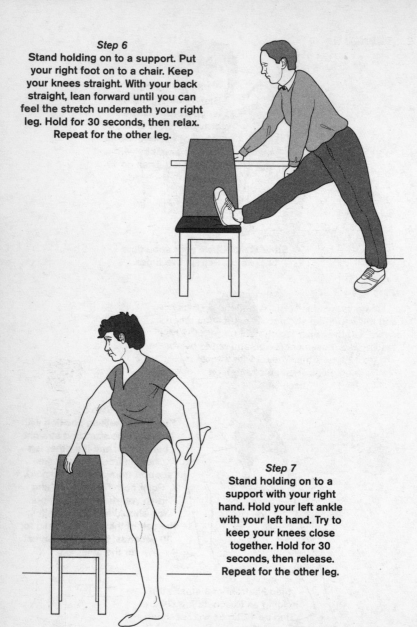

Step 6
Stand holding on to a support. Put your right foot on to a chair. Keep your knees straight. With your back straight, lean forward until you can feel the stretch underneath your right leg. Hold for 30 seconds, then relax. Repeat for the other leg.

Step 7
Stand holding on to a support with your right hand. Hold your left ankle with your left hand. Try to keep your knees close together. Hold for 30 seconds, then release. Repeat for the other leg.

2. STRENGTH

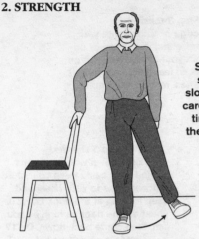

Step 1 (easier)
Stand holding on to a support. Lift your leg slowly out to the side (be careful not to twist). Do 12 times, then repeat with the other leg. Then do 12 more on each side.

Step 1 (harder)
Lie on your side. Keep the bottom leg bent and the upper leg straight. Keep the hips rolled forward. Lift the upper leg straight up with the heel leading the movement (be careful not to twist). Do 12 times, then repeat with the other leg. Rest. Then do 12 more on each side.

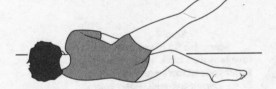

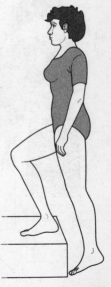

Step 2
Stand in front of a small step, holding on to something secure. Step up 12 times with each leg. Rest and repeat.

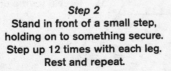

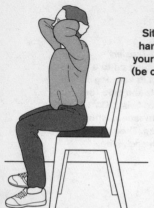

Step 3 (easier)
Sit on the edge of a chair with your hands either behind your head or on your hips. Arch your back, then let it go (be careful not to lean back or forward). Do 12 times, rest and repeat.

Step 3 (harder)
Lie face down with your arms behind your back. Keep your chin down close to your chest and keep looking at the floor. Lift your chest off the floor as high as you can, then come back down. Do 12 times, rest and repeat.

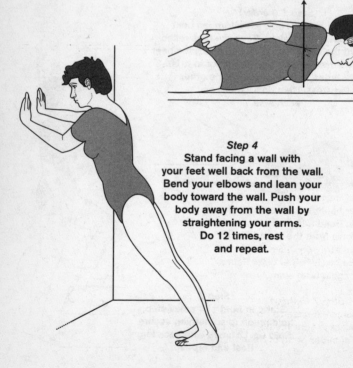

Step 4
Stand facing a wall with your feet well back from the wall. Bend your elbows and lean your body toward the wall. Push your body away from the wall by straightening your arms. Do 12 times, rest and repeat.

Step 5
Stand up and sit down without using your hands for two minutes.

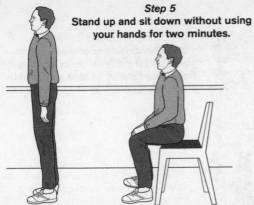

Step 6
Stand and hold on to a support. Rise up on to your toes, and then lower. Do 12 times, rest and repeat.

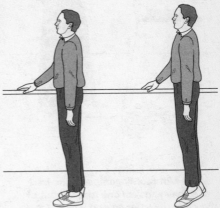

Step 7 (easier)
Hang your hands over the edge of a chair back. Bend and flex your hands up and down from the wrists. Do 12 times, then turn your hands over and do 12 more on the other side. Repeat again both sides.

Step 7 (harder)
Do the same exercise as above but hold a weight in your hands, such as a bag of sugar or tin of beans.

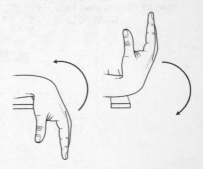

3. BALANCE

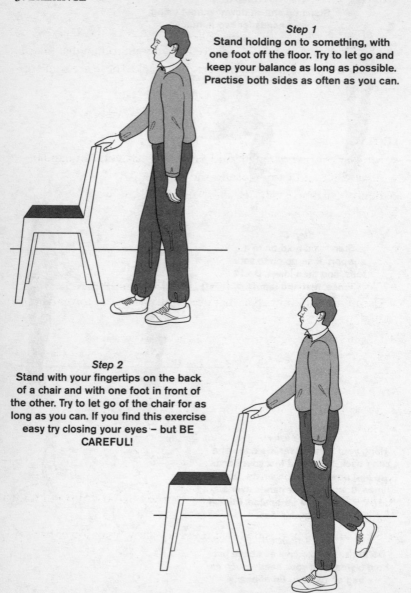

Step 1
Stand holding on to something, with one foot off the floor. Try to let go and keep your balance as long as possible. Practise both sides as often as you can.

Step 2
Stand with your fingertips on the back of a chair and with one foot in front of the other. Try to let go of the chair for as long as you can. If you find this exercise easy try closing your eyes – but BE CAREFUL!

Taking care of your back

The spine is one of the most common areas of the body to be affected by osteoporosis. It is therefore very important that people suffering from osteoporosis protect their back. These are some tips for doing so.

LIFTING
- Know your own strength and only lift what you can handle.
- Always lift and carry close to the body.
- Bend your knees and let your legs do all the work.
- Don't twist your back – turn with your feet.

SITTING
- Avoid low soft chairs that have poor back support.
- Use an upright firm chair that does not allow your lower back to slouch.
- Get up and straighten your back every 30 minutes.

STANDING
- Avoid bending forwards for long periods of time.
- Have your working surface at a comfortable height.

DRIVING
- Have frequent breaks during long journeys to stand up and walk around a little.
- Sit in an upright position that does not allow your lower back to slouch.

SLEEPING

- Using a firm mattress will give your back more support.
- Getting into bed:
  - ☐ Sit at the side of the bed
  - ☐ Lower yourself on to your elbow
  - ☐ Lower further on to your shoulder, bending your knees at the same time
  - ☐ Draw your knees up until your legs are on the bed
  - ☐ Roll your body and knees together to face the ceiling.
- Reverse this sequence to get out of bed.

Appendix D

Calcium Content of Common Foods

A daily intake of 1000mg (milligrams) of calcium by adults supplies the body's daily needs and helps to maintain bone strength. Although dairy products are the best-known sources of calcium many non-dairy products are also good. The following is a small selection of common foods. Your GP can refer you to a dietician if you need more detailed advice.

Food group	Example	Portion size	Milligrams of calcium per portion
Dairy	Milk (all types)	200ml glass	240
	Ice cream	60g / 2oz	60
	Plain yoghurt	125g pot	250
	Fruit yoghurt	125g pot	170
	Hard cheese (e.g. Cheddar)	30g / 1oz	225
	Soft cheese (e.g. Brie)	30g / 1oz	80
Bread	White	One slice	30
	Wholemeal	One slice	9
Crackers	Cream crackers	2	18
	Ryvita	2	8
Flour	Soya	1 heaped tbsp	63
	White	1 heaped tbsp	46
	Wholemeal	1 heaped tbsp	11
Sweet	Fully coated in chocolate, e.g. Club	1	26
	Chocolate digestive	1	14
Cereals	Ready Brek	130g	84
	Muesli	70g	77
	All Bran	50g	34
	Weetabix	1	7
	Cornflakes	40g	3
Pulses	Baked beans	2 tbsp	54
	Vegetable soup (thick)	250ml bowl	42
	Chick peas	2 tbsp	24
	Lentils	2 tbsp	6

Food group	Example	Portion size	Milligrams of calcium per portion
Nuts	Almonds	6 whole	25
	Brazils	3 whole	18
	Peanuts	Small bag (25g)	15
Fruits	Dried figs	40g	92
	Rhubarb, stewed	Small bowl	49
	Blackberries	Small bowl	49
	Orange	1 small	43
	Raspberries	15	15
	Raisins	1 tbsp	14
	Dried apricots	2	12
	Dried dates	2	11
Vegetables	Spinach	80g	128
	Cabbage, boiled	90g	48
	Broccoli tops	100g	40
	Turnip, boiled	60g	27
	Celery, boiled	50g	25
	Carrots, boiled	60g	21
	Leeks	80g	16
Meat & meat products	Gammon	170g	42
	Marmite	1 heaped tsp	22
	Oxo	1 cube	13
	Meat paste	Sandwich portion	10

Food group	Example	Portion size	Milligrams of calcium per portion
Fish	Whitebait, fried	80g	700
	Sardines, tinned	Sandwich portion	230
	Pilchards, tinned	50g	150
	Prawns	60g	140
	Shrimps	50g	64
Miscellaneous	Tofu	100g	139
	Fruit gums	Tube (33g)	121
	Tortilla chips	30g	45
	Spaghetti, tinned	2 tbsp	19